# Study Skills for Nursing and Midwifery Students

**Philip A. Scullion and David A. Guest**

Open University Press

Open University Press
McGraw-Hill Education
McGraw-Hill House
Shoppenhangers Road
Maidenhead
Berkshire
England
SL6 2QL

email: enquiries@openup.co.uk
world wide web: www.openup.co.uk

and Two Penn Plaza, New York, NY 10121-2289, USA

First published 2007
Reprinted 2010

A catalogue record of this book is available from the British Library

ISBN-10: 0 335 22220 X (pb)   0 335 22221 8 (hb)
ISBN-13: 978 0 335 22220 9 (pb)   978 0 335 22221 6 (hb)

Library of Congress Cataloguing-in-Publication Data
CIP data applied for

Typeset by RefineCatch Limited, Bungay, Suffolk
Printed in UK by Ashford Colour Press Ltd, Gosport, Hants.

The McGraw-Hill Companies

# Study Skills for Nursing and Midwifery Students

# Contents

*Series editor's preface*                                                    vii

**Part 1 The student nurse and midwife as a novice learner**

1 Engaging with university learning                                            3

2 Taking control of yourself: nurses and midwives as learners                21

3 Making information work for nursing and midwifery students                 36

**Part 2 Beginning to develop effective study skills**

4 Strategies for successful learning in nursing and midwifery                57

5 Reflective learning in clinical practice                                   78

**Part 3 Becoming competent: advanced learning for nursing and midwifery students**

6 Literature searching skills for midwives and nurses                       101

7 Proficient use of evidence and research to support nursing and
  midwifery                                                                 120

**Part 4 Demonstrating proficiency through assessment**

8 Critical analysis and higher-level skills for nurses and midwives         145

9 Coping with examinations and assessments                                  161

**Part 5 Expertise for success: the lifelong learner in nursing and midwifery**

10  Career pathways in nursing and midwifery                    183

11  Lifelong learning organizations and CPD to sustain your
     professional practice                                      190

*References*                                                     209
*Glossary*                                                       216
*Index*                                                          219

# Series editor's preface

*Study Skills* cover all those abilities that make it possible to cope with the demands of academic and professional pursuits. For people just embarking on a course of study they include being able to deal with all the intellectual, emotional and social challenges that are part of the day-to-day demands of being a student. Beyond the skills involved in coping are those that enable students to do well in their chosen disciplines. These embrace much more than the ability to memorize or understand the topics of study, reaching into time management, ethics and the personal and interpersonal upheavals that are often such an important part of the student's life.

The study skills that are mastered at university, or for some people earlier when studying at school, are central to what everyone has to offer as a graduate and/or professional. Some people would even suggest that the main contribution of a university degree is to provide a person with the skills for studying. It is these skills that will help the person through the rest of their career.

Studying is a skill that can be mastered like many others, by first understanding the process then by developing appropriate habits through active involvement. Yet whilst there are some aspects of the process that are common to all forms of study there are often important facets of any particular area of study that demand special skills. Further, even when the skills may be relevant across a number of different disciplines it is usually easier to understand what is required by embedding consideration of them within the specific topic.

This series of books is therefore being published with guidance on how to be an effective student within each of a series of specific domains. By dealing with study skills in relation to the area of study it is possible to ensure that the examples are directly pertinent to the student of that area, rather than being general exhortations. The books thus complement the many other publications available on such general topics as essay writing or taking examinations.

The focus on particular areas of study also enables the authors to follow the particular educational trajectory from the early entry into college or university right through to becoming a recognised professional in the chosen discipline. It allows the authors to draw on examples that speak directly to students about issues in their own lives. It also enables the books to identify particular topics that are of special significance for any given discipline.

This series therefore provides a valuable resource to all students that they can draw on as a friend and guide throughout their course of study and beyond.

David Canter
Series Editor
University of Liverpool

# Part 1

The student nurse and midwife as a novice learner

# 1

# Engaging with university learning

*Introduction • Subject content • Study skills: the process of learning
• Registration on a course • Ice-breakers • What the university expects
• Relationships • Methods of teaching and learning • Getting the best from
your course • Engaging in established quality systems • Referencing
• Conclusions*

Efforts spent engaging with the university and developing your study skills will make your nursing or midwifery course so much more of a pleasure.

This chapter sets out to help you settle into university learning, and introduce you to changes and challenges, so that you can become actively engaged with the educational and other experiences the course will expose you to. If you immerse yourself in the course, the experience of being at university and the study possibilities, you are likely to be more than just successful. You are likely to enjoy your studies and develop habits and attitudes that will enhance your learning well beyond completing the course. 'A higher education experience is not a commodity, it is a participatory experience' (Harvey 2006:15); research by Forbes and Spence (1991) indicates that the quality of your engagement in learning tasks is key to learning. Your engagement with the university and the learning opportunities it offers directly impacts on your progress and success.

# Introduction

By now you will probably have been officially welcomed to the university by some very senior person such as the Dean, a professor or a head of department, in an impressive lecture theatre. You may already have felt a twinge of underlying anxiety that often accompanies change or new experiences. Ten years ago most people entering nursing or midwifery would not have envisaged going to university but these subjects are now firmly located in university departments or faculties where they make up a major proportion of student numbers.

Yet a degree or diploma may not be your main purpose. You may simply wish to extend your career as a qualified nurse or midwife by undertaking additional learning or, more likely, you are in year one of a three-year course which will lead to an initial qualification in nursing or midwifery. In either case you may feel very much the novice as a student in the university setting. However there are many people within the university and practice settings, often older, experienced nurses or midwives who are willing to assist you in a fairly smooth transition into university life as pointed out by Watson *et al.* (2006) in a national survey. You are in good company.

Some aspects of studying at university are very different from school, college or the workplace. This is especially noticeable if you have been out of education for a few years. Most nurses and midwives, or nursing and midwifery students, do not start a university course directly from school or college. Your university is aware that many of its students are mature and so have particular needs.

Work at university can be divided into the 'subject content' which focuses on the knowledge you gain about the subjects related to nursing or midwifery and 'process' which relates to the ways in which you gain that specific content and demonstrate this as evidence of your learning.

# Subject content

During your course or module you will pursue knowledge and understanding, and develop cognitive, practical and transferable skills related to the world of your selected branch of nursing or midwifery. Professional values and attitudes will also be developed through theoretical and practical learning opportunities and experiences, though these may be less explicit in teaching and assessments.

While some 'subject content' will be valuable across all courses and disciplines, and indeed you will share some modules with students from other courses, much of it is quite specific to your own course. It is however likely to include the following areas:

- the theoretical basis of your defined area of practice, e.g.
  - anatomy and physiology
  - applied psychology and sociology
  - legal and ethical issues
  - pathophysiology
  - pharmacology
  - therapeutic interventions
- current issues in the context of health care practice
- evidence-based practice, research and its application to practice
- strategies for assisting individual clients in the changing context of health care environments
- theoretical ideas which underpin practice
- using information from a variety of sources in order to gain a coherent understanding of theory and practice
- working as part of an inter-professional team
- career opportunities and challenges ahead; beginning to plan a career path.

The acquisition of the subject content will move you along the continuum from 'novice to expert' in nursing or midwifery considerably, as described by Patricia Benner (1984).

## Study skills: the process of learning

Whilst this book draws on a range of examples from relevant subject content its main focus is on the processes. You will need to engage with these processes in order to successfully master the necessary content, gain competency and pass the assessments in both theory and practice. Clearly you have much to contribute to the learning process but taking you from novice to expert in terms of the processes involved in study and learning will mean engaging with university learning in many of the following areas:

- taking control of yourself, motivation and organization
- information technology and using the library
- developing strategies for successful learning
- reflective learning from practice placements
- becoming competent in literature searching

- proficient use of evidence and research
- demonstrating critical analysis and higher-level skills
- expertise for success in selected career pathways
- continuing professional development and becoming a lifelong learner.

The ways in which you learn the specific content varies but will include:

- a wide range of teaching methods, e.g.
  - lecture, seminar, group work
- developing and using skills, e.g.
  - information seeking
  - reading effectively
  - note taking from many sources
  - understanding academic language
  - managing time and prioritizing workloads
- understanding and becoming proficient in:
  - essay and report writing
  - referencing sources used
  - research methods
- confidently managing:
  - working as part of an inter-professional team
  - presenting information to colleagues orally, in writing and electronically
  - revision
  - examinations and other assessments
  - dissertation.

Becoming skilled in *studying* is often overlooked by students. Some of the activities listed above will obviously require you to develop skills such as 'information seeking' via the library and the internet. Others such as revision or seminar work will be far less obvious. Yet in all of these, developing study skills can make your performance more expert, require less effort and will result in gaining far more from activities compared with a friend who has not made the effort to become skilled as a student.

Overall, if you become skilled at the processes of learning you will develop independence and be able to take responsibility for lifelong learning and your own professional development. You will advance as a student from 'novice to expert' too. Students who take note of the need to learn the processes and not just the content work efficiently and more effectively. Developing your study skills for success will move you from an indecisive novice beginner to a confident, independent, efficient student with expertise in many of the processes of learning.

# Registration on a course

This is boring but essential. Be prepared to patiently produce documents, fill in forms, sign declarations, sit in front of a digital camera for your ID card, and ensure that details are all correct. Always use your full correct name in the correct order. Your attention to detail will avoid delays and problems at a later date and if there are big queues or spare time you can use it to get to know some of your new colleagues.

Registering for the correct course and completing all the documentation is vital for:

- access to university library and computer systems
- communications from different university departments
- ensuring you appear on official module and course lists
- invoicing for modules and courses, accommodation and fees
- personal details on awards
- physical access to facilities
- receiving your bursary
- receiving your invitation to the award ceremony
- confirming details with the Nursing and Midwifery Council which maintains the register of nursing and midwifery qualifications.

# Ice-breakers

Some ice-breakers chill my spine! You may be cajoled into participating in ice-breaker activities designed to facilitate the process of getting to know people who are newly brought together in a group: your cohort of students and associated staff. These take various forms from drinking coffee and mingling in a socially conducive setting to the more bizarre 'games' where you are required to characterize yourself as an animal of your choice! The intentions are good and indeed the sooner you do begin to form working relationships and friendship groups, the better. Relationships will inevitably shift and develop as the course progresses since it is unlikely that the person whom the seating arrangement places you near on day one would have been your first choice companion for three or more years. For pre-registration courses the overall group numbers will be large so it is impractical to become study buddies with them all but you really should make an effort to establish healthy working relationships and friendships with several people.

Even if ice-breakers are not your favourite pastime, small groups are popular and will be used within the course, so do take the opportunities as they arise, or create your own. One way of beginning this process is to join with others, perhaps between four and ten people, in the following exercise.

## Exercise 1.1

This simply asks you to spend some time thinking about Challenges, Concerns and Contributions. Individually or in a group compile three lists:

1 Challenges: in anticipation of the course, based on your current understanding, note the things you are likely to find challenging. Remember many people thrive on challenges and these may be positive, such as the challenge to develop the confidence to cope in an emergency situation.
2 Concerns: here you should concentrate on those things that may provoke slight anxiety based on your understanding of the demands of the course. Make a list identifying causes of your main concerns.
3 Contributions: this may need more time and thought and typically produces the shortest list. However, this need not be so. Think about your experiences and achievements in all aspects of your life. Consider how these have prepared you for nursing or midwifery and the particular course you are registered on. You may feel the need to consult family members, friends or work colleagues as others may have more insight into your strengths than you have. The aim is to devise a list of attributes, skills, knowledge or attitudes which will contribute to success on the course for you and others.

### Challenges

If you can, discuss these with colleagues and in particular identify where and how these challenges may be met and what support may be necessary to help in their achievement. Jot down questions that remain unanswered.

### Concerns

Mingled with the excitement, you will naturally be concerned about some issues and it is wise to identify these and deal with them at an early stage. Many adult learners will begin to feel a lack of confidence in their own abilities particularly as the demands of the course become apparent. Other issues or common concerns reported by student groups at the beginning of courses include:

• an undisturbed place to study
• availability of tutorial staff

- being away from home
- finances
- finding materials for study
- level of difficulty
- level of support available
- other commitment, e.g. child care
- overall workload
- particular weaknesses, e.g. academic writing, client-related fears
- risk of failure at exams.

Discuss items on your list with others and allow them to express their concerns. Then move the conversation on to possible solutions or strategies to avoid the issue getting to the stage of becoming a real problem. In a small group there is likely to be someone who has experience in coping with these or similar concerns. Share ideas, and even jot down things which appear to have potential to assist you. Also jot down concerns or questions that remain unanswered.

Near the beginning of a course or module many of these issues will be addressed explicitly, perhaps during Freshers' Week or an induction day. However, much of what is presented soon becomes a hazy memory so do file most of the paperwork so that when an issue arises a few months into the course you will be able to locate the detail you need. Even if you cannot there are several easy ways of locating course-related details to answer your specific questions.

You may try:

- other students on your course
- course-specific notice board
- reception staff
- faculty or school student support office
- personal tutor
- course director
- module leader
- university website
- the student union.

And if all else fails the university will have a large centralised department often called 'Student Services' which perhaps should have been your first port of call. They will direct your questions to the appropriate person or department and provide help with things like:

- essential needs
  - accommodation
  - catering

  o funding (e.g. NHS bursaries)
  o medical services (e.g. local GP)
- specialist advice
  o chaplaincy
  o counselling
  o employment opportunities while a student
  o disabilities office
  o dyslexia
- directions to
  o learning and study support
  o mental health support services
  o nursery
  o sports
  o welfare and hardship
  o careers guidance.

Anything left on your list of jottings may form the basis for one of your first tutorials.

## Contributions

Everyone will have different starting points on a course and their contributions to their own and group learning will vary accordingly. With the average age of pre-registration students being around 29 (Royal College of Nursing, 2004) undoubtedly a typical group of pre-registration students is made up of those with a multitude of family and career experiences and associated expertise. Qualified nurses or midwives undertaking continuing professional development (CPD) courses will similarly have many skills and much knowledge and experience which is transferable to their new student status.

A key distinguishing feature at the start of pre-registration courses may exist between the school leaver and the mature entrant. Each group typically feels disadvantaged in comparison with the other. Desirable characteristics assumed to be associated with these are listed in Table 1.1.

These typifications, if true for individuals, will certainly be helpful in some circumstances. Over time however they balance each other out so that neither group is disadvantaged, and where working friendships emerge between the mature and the school leaver entrant, each group will benefit from sharing skill sets. Irrespective of your starting point, do not underestimate the fact that you, and your new peers, have a lot that will help you cope with the changes and meet the challenges you currently face, more so if you make a conscious decision to offer and receive mutual support.

**Table 1.1** Assumed characteristics of students

| School leaver | Mature entrant |
|---|---|
| Confidence as a student | Confidence as a person |
| IT literate | Life experiences |
| Proficient at studying | Personal or family illness or childrearing experience |
| Recent experience of courses and exams | Able to deal with children |
| Lots of spare time | Practical skills, especially if experience working in |
| Few outside responsibilities | health care |

# What the university expects

The ethos is different from school. You are expected to be self-motivated and once work is set few will check up on you. Once your work is submitted there are no opportunities to resubmit in order to gain additional marks. Deadlines for coursework are set and exam schedules are published; beyond these dates penalties are imposed if they are missed.

## On campus and in placement

There are university-wide regulations but you may be asked to be involved in drawing up agreements about expectations within the faculty. These are designed to promote participation and mutual respect amongst peers and between peers and staff. For some the nuisance value of mobile phones, including (irritating) text messaging, attendance and promptness will be key issues which may hinder group learning if not addressed. Any such rules will be well publicised and they can be used in exceptional circumstances to challenge unacceptable behaviours. Certain professional expectations are enshrined in the Nursing and Midwifery Council Code of Conduct (2004a) and in advance of registering a qualification the university will be asked to provide a declaration of good character (Nursing and Midwifery Order 2001). If there are serious issues your university may exclude students from the course on the grounds of professional unsuitability. A mature approach however will ensure that behaviour is generally professional and conducive to learning.

# Relationships

Establishing good relationships and communications with key people and departments in a huge organization, such as a university and its associated NHS and other health care providers, will make the course that much easier. These may be formal:

- academic supervisor
- course administrator
- course director
- library staff
- link tutor
- mentor
- module leader
- practice facilitator
- secretarial staff who deal with bursaries or manage the diary of academic staff
- staff within placements

or largely informal:

- peers
- personal tutor
- university reception staff
- staff who receive and distribute coursework
- students from other groups
- students on related courses, e.g. physiotherapy, medicine, clinical psychology, social work
- technicians who provide IT support within the university.

These and many others will have some relationship with you or your work and you may need to obtain their assistance at various points in the course. You will need to respect and appreciate their roles and responsibilities to ensure your engagement is as productive as possible. Most pressing however will be your experience of the actual teaching and how you and your peers engage with this for effective learning.

# Methods of teaching and learning

Most students would expect the course to have lectures and seminars and provide opportunities to develop a wide range of practical skills, mainly in placements.

However, nursing and midwifery students will be exposed to a wide variety of methods of teaching and learning, some of which may take you out of your comfort zone.

## Exercise 1.2

• Think about your most recent experience of undertaking a course, study day or school
• Try to list all the methods of teaching you were exposed to
• Add to that list methods you have heard of but have no direct experience of
• Of these identify those you encountered most frequently
• Identify which is the one you are MOST and LEAST comfortable with
• Try to list a few reasons explaining your preferences

Clearly there are approaches to teaching that suit you. Perhaps the method you identified as most comfortable is the one you have been exposed to most. However, this may not be the most effective and if you engage only with the methods you are comfortable with your experience at university will be limited, especially on a nursing or midwifery course. Some subjects lend themselves to effective delivery by lecture and these will form a key part of your academic experience. However, if you identified role-play amongst your least favourite methods, you are in very good company. But if organized and handled well, role-play can provide powerful learning opportunities, invaluable when applied to real patient care situations.

# Getting the best from your course

The range of methods employed will provide something for everyone, but it is important for you to make sure that you make the most of every opportunity. I have sat through lectures and occasionally the group consensus was 'what an utter waste of time!' You may experience this occasionally but often you have the ability to make lectures and other forms of learning more effective. So if you enter with a closed mind, for example determined that you hate debates, then your attitude may just make debates a non-event for you and their quality will be diminished for your group because of your withdrawal.

What follows (Table 1.2) is a list of the types of educational experiences you will encounter within the confines of the university. Some of them form essential prerequisites for any learning that may occur in practice. For instance pre-registration students must demonstrate basic competence in skills such as

**Table 1.2** Range of educational methods

| Method | Main features | Getting the best from this method |
| --- | --- | --- |
| Lecture | Topics are introduced to large groups by a formal presentation, often with limited interaction between lecturer and students<br><br>These are frequently supported by a PowerPoint presentation<br><br>Lecture programmes will often be supplemented with appropriate required reading | Prepare by looking at the title of the lecture in advance and explore the meanings of new terminology<br><br>Do some advance reading that may be suggested in course documents to provide an overview<br><br>Ensure you are alert and on time, perhaps arriving early to get a reasonable seat<br><br>Bring the necessary equipment and develop your note taking skills<br><br>Jot down questions, often they are welcomed during or at the end of the lecture<br><br>Do not hesitate to stay back to explore things further with the lecturer unless they are obviously in a hurry<br><br>PowerPoint presentation or lecture notes are usually freely available to students in electronic format<br><br>Follow up with further reading as required and attend to your notes with particular attention to the session objectives |
| Seminar | Topic orientated and take the form of a presentation by lecturers, individual students or small groups of students<br><br>The style may be informal and one key aim is to allocate around one-third of the available time for discussion since critical comment and discussion form an integral part of a seminar<br><br>This is a method often used for both learning and assessment | This approach can be very productive and stimulating for learning and exposing your knowledge or attitude 'gaps'<br><br>If you are presenting the key is preparation, so ensure you over-prepare<br><br>If this is a group effort meet with others to negotiate roles and responsibilities<br><br>When speaking you cover much more than anticipated in the allotted time<br><br>Decide on any communication aid e.g. flip chart, poster, PowerPoint and check their availability<br><br>Be prepared for silence when you ask 'Any questions?' by bringing thought-provoking statements and possibly slightly controversial questions to pose<br><br>Write some notes soon after your seminar and follow up queries that were not fully exhausted; you may have to present a write-up for marking!<br><br>Where the seminar involves mixed disciplines use these to consider an inter-professional perspective |

If you were not the presenter remember being 'active' promotes your own learning; be willing to discuss the topic and do some reading and thinking in advance

| Tutorials | A discussion session which is chaired by a member of staff and consists of any number of students from one to approximately twenty<br><br>Used to discuss new concepts being introduced in lectures and issues that emerge solely from the student's own agenda | One-to-one tutorials are less likely to be offered, but much can be gained from the participation of peers<br><br>Attend promptly and after preparing properly<br><br>Mobile phones have many uses but not in tutorials<br><br>Remain focused, the lecturer is likely to have a whole list of groups and will not have time to waste or go beyond the time allocated<br><br>If the topic is open, or the agenda is yours to determine, ensure you have some key issues or questions to discuss<br><br>Take a few notes and do follow-up on suggestions made, e.g. to introduce a new perspective (such as patients' wishes regarding the provision of information prior to surgery), or read certain named articles |
| Role-play | An imaginable but fictional situation is presented and you will typically be given an outline of the role you are required to take on<br><br>The session may be video-recorded for later analysis by yourself or a wider audience<br><br>Sometimes used for assessment<br><br>Requires small groups where trust is established between members | Carefully read any instructions and discuss the remit with the session leader<br><br>Do not instantly dismiss this as unrealistic, give it a fair chance<br><br>To act out situations may be safer than meeting them in reality for the first time<br><br>Be prepared to support the facilitator and colleagues, a mature approach will add value to this method<br><br>While you are attempting to use empathy in engaging with the role-play this may develop as part of the post-role-play analysis<br><br>Discuss the extent to which this has prepared you for a real clinical encounter similar to the role-play scenario<br><br>Ensure that you and other participants involved are clear that role-play requires people to take on the role of other people; participants were not being themselves!<br><br>Review the learning and learning deficits this may have revealed and consider writing a reflective account in your portfolio |

(*Continued overleaf*)

**Table 1.2** Continued

| Method | Main features | Getting the best from this method |
| --- | --- | --- |
| Web-based learning/ projects | These may form a major component in some courses<br><br>They vary greatly but consist of interactive material presented via computer, often a system such as 'Web-CT'<br><br>Patient scenarios may be included using video clips<br><br>You will be expected to participate, contribute to discussion forums and submit work in the form of tests, quizzes, reports or essays via an electronic Internet-based platform | Take time to undertake any suggested preparations such as a launch event or online PowerPoint presentation<br><br>Read and abide by the university policy covering the use of computers<br><br>Make sure you are clear about your role; some aspects of web-based learning will usually be assessed<br><br>Understand whether your submissions are public (like a discussion board) or private (like e-mail)<br><br>Check any work carefully before you upload it to the web-based site as your errors may cause embarrassment; usually only key lecturers have the authority to alter or delete your submissions<br><br>Make sure you are polite and concise in any submissions and ensure they can be clearly linked to previous submissions (threads) where appropriate<br><br>If you are allocated to groups keep in touch regularly with other group members – the IT system will make this easy to achieve<br><br>May follow the format of an online seminar in virtual time involving members of the inter-professional team<br><br>N.B. Your lecturers will have an electronic log of ALL your interaction within these sites (except where there is an e-mail function which remains private) and there may be a minimum requirement for participation |
| Problem-based learning | An instructional method involving small groups or teams used to gain knowledge and problem-solving skills. Here the problem is presented via 'triggers' before the relevant material has been learned (Wilkie 2000:11) | Take note of the 'triggers', which may be written scenarios, photographs or video clips and brainstorm with the team to identify gaps in knowledge<br><br>Discuss the areas where pertinent information is required in order to identify/solve the problem/s<br><br>Ensure good team working and be clear about your accepted responsibilities; and deliver the goods!<br><br>Be supportive of your team members<br><br>Some find this approach difficult to engage with as it leaves uncertainties but try to reserve judgements on this method until well after the completion of the tasks |

| | | |
|---|---|---|
| Formal debate | A 'chair' and two teams are required | Volunteer to join the panel if the opportunity arises |
| | A clear statement is devised: the 'motion', which should be published in advance | If not do some advance reading around the motion and if possible form an opinion |
| | | Be open to listen to both sides and put your questions through the chair to panel members |
| | Outside speakers may be invited to take these roles but if students do so they may be obliged to argue against their own personal convictions | This method has the potential to sharpen your critical-thinking skills on matters related to ethics, attitudes and values |
| | | Allows you to see things from a different perspective and even if your views are not altered during the course of the debate you will gain valuable insights |
| | | N.B. Some panel members may have been arguing against their personal convictions |
| Guided study | Printed or online guide which is lecturer-directed | These are likely to be clearly linked to the outcome of a course or module and may form an essential integral part of the learning required |
| | Involves students seeking information on specific topics designed to enable further development of knowledge and critical thinking | Read the instructions carefully and do not hesitate to seek clarification from lecturers |
| | | Determine if the activities and outcomes could be best achieved by collaborating with selected colleagues; if so form a team |
| | These may be incorporated into the timetable for the purpose of feedback and discussion aimed at sharing and consolidating learning | Feedback opportunities are important to ensure learning has been accurate and no key points are missed, so use them fully |
| Simulation | The situation may be similar to role-play but you assume your own identity. The situation consists of a scenario in a classroom or clinical laboratory, possibly using a mannequin (SIM MAN) | The great benefit here is that you act in-role, as a nurse or midwife (student) and practise clinical skills and decision making |
| | | The more you engage with this the more potential for learning |
| | Useful to simulate cardiac or other physiological disturbances and provide rapid feedback | Provides opportunities for team work, rehearsing emergencies and learning where the 'patient' is an expensive mannequin rather than a priceless human being! |
| | | Important to reflect on this experience preferably within the team involved |

moving and handling in a skills laboratory before being allowed to proceed to clinical placements. By actively engaging in each of these as you encounter them, you will be able to exploit them fully for their educational value both in terms of subject content and skills and competence in the processes of learning.

## Exercise 1.3

Consider those methods you like and review whether your own approach could be made even more effective, for example skim-reading prior to a lecture. Select ONE method that you are unfamiliar with or dislike.

- Make a special effort to engage with this method at the next opportunity
- Reflect on your experiences and discuss these with student friends or academic staff

Match the following topics with a suitable method of teaching and learning:

1  cardiopulmonary resuscitation
2  stigma associated with learning disability or mental health
3  the anatomy of the nervous system
4  the Children Act and its implications for children's nursing services
5  assessment and detection of domestic violence during pregnancy.

It may be clear that the most effective methods in each of these examples pro-vided will differ and in order to get the best from the course appropriate matching of methods to topics will be necessary. As a student you will do well to extend your repertoire and embrace many of these methods.

# Engaging in established quality systems

Your university has a commitment to providing an excellent service and this will be made explicit in its mission statement. While you may sail through your course without any knowledge of this, the aspiration to provide excellence needs to be checked and who better to consult than you? Directly or indirectly it is students who pay towards the running of universities and your views on the nature and quality of its provision are important and will be sought. The course or module leaders need to know how well their plans are being delivered. You will be given feedback on your performance and the university certainly needs feedback from you. This is most frequently requested via evaluation questionnaires or other methods at the end of modules or placements.

Other formal mechanisms will be in place such as a system where several student representatives from each course intake will meet senior university staff periodically to share information and raise issues of concern. In addition to this, where new courses are being planned there will be invitations for students to contribute views. Courses where the NHS or other bodies are stakeholders will have regular meetings with key senior academic staff and managers and often there is a constitutional requirement for students' views to be represented. Actually putting yourself forward on to some of these groups will have positive benefits to you; it will help you to network and develop communication and other skills.

- Get to know which issues are taken to which groups or meetings
- Consider becoming a group representative
- Liaise with your representatives and ensure you are kept well informed; this is likely to involve keeping an eye on the appropriate notice board or website
- Do not hesitate to ask your student representatives to bring issues for commendation or concern to their regular meetings

If there are areas of excellence and you have benefited from these it will help if you voice your views. More important, perhaps, if there are concerns or inadequacies, unless you voice these they are unlikely to improve and they may have a negative effect on the quality of your learning opportunities. A mature approach is required, systems to deal with such issues exist, and you may need to be specific about the circumstances. If you have suggestions that may be feasible to improve conditions or solve problems they are likely to be well received.

# Referencing

While you are expected to use sources of information, essentially the work you produce, such as an essay, must be your own work. Your university will provide guidance on working with others, collusion, cheating and plagiarism. Plagiarism is classed as a form of cheating and is discussed more fully in Chapter 9, but 'many studies show that the bulk of plagiarism can be attributed to students who do not understand academic requirements' (Joint Information Systems Committee, 2005). In view of this you will need to become familiar with referencing.

This consists of a system of using and listing the sources you have used in an academic piece of work, for example an essay, report or reflective account of practice. One of the key functions of any referencing system is to enable students to accurately attribute ideas to their original sources. In making such a clear statement you may avoid the possibility of naïve plagiarism. There are a number of referencing systems, the commonest in nursing and midwifery is the Harvard system. Most universities will have their own particular version of the Harvard system. While others have written in detail on this topic (Gopee, 1999), here you are advised to become familiar with the particular version approved by your university.

### Key elements of the Harvard referencing system

- Provides instructions on the detail required in text, i.e. the body of your essay and the alphabetical list required at the end of your work
- Demonstrates precisely how to use 'quotations' or citations in the text of your assignments
- In the text usually just the author's surname and the year of publication are required often in brackets (surname, year)
- Distinguishes between books, journal articles, websites and other sources
- Makes a distinction between a reference list and a bibliography
- Prescribes the order in which detail should be presented within these lists
- Prescribes the use of punctuation, *italics*, **bold** or underlining

It may be quite alien to read text which is frequently interrupted by authors' surnames and years, more so to get used to writing using this style of referencing. An alternative referencing system is the Vancouver system. This system will be found in some journals and uses numbers in the text, usually in superscript with the detail provided on a list at the end of the article or essay.

The exact detail is best discovered from your own university course handbook or website but it is an academic convention that you must rapidly get to grips with. In year one your lecturers may be lenient but by year three failure to adhere to the system in operation is likely to lose you marks.

# Conclusions

University will present a challenge to many nursing and midwifery students. This challenge represents positive opportunities to engage with the methods of teaching and learning and the array of departments and people who play a key collaborative role in helping you to make your student experience a success. Midwifery and nursing are rapidly developing professions: the subject content of ten years ago will not meet the needs of today's clients. Experience mingled with up-to-date knowledge and skills are vital and a commitment to lifelong learning is rapidly becoming the norm. By becoming more expert in the processes of learning you will develop independence and confidence as a student; this is vital to enable your practice to be evidence based. Engagement in learning therefore reflects commitment to patient care today and into the future.

# 2

# Taking control of yourself: nurses and midwives as learners

*Introduction • Nurses and midwives as learners • Who is in control? • Locus of control • Are you really helpless? • Choosing study friends • Ground rules • Emotional control • Motivation • Goals • Resources • Capturing time • The three D's • Taking control of your timetable • Conclusions*

This chapter examines who controls your learning, 'locus of control' and feelings of helplessness which are sometimes associated with learning. Being strategic and developing relationships with 'study friends', taking control of your emotions, motivation and time management are also covered. It will encourage you not only to see the benefits of taking control of yourself but also to actually assume command of your own studies. Ideally you should read this chapter at an early stage in your course, but if you have drifted along aimlessly being influenced by external pressures like a rudderless ship, the ideas here can help you recover some lost ground and reinstate you as your own captain.

## Introduction

Equipped with a more realistic idea of the requirements of a university-based nursing or midwifery course and determined to make the most of it, you are now faced with the task of putting these ideas and aspirations into practice. You may be convinced that to be fully engaged with a wide range of approaches to learning is helpful. However, developing competence in the processes of learning and establishing fruitful working relationships with new people will not just happen. You need to seize the opportunities, plan, organize, keep tabs on progress, review and prioritize. You need to assume responsibility for your own learning and deliberately take control of your situation.

> A man who tried to win a game, but did not even know the aim,
> Came last, completely missed the goal, because he did not take control.
>
> (Anon)

## Nurses and midwives as learners

Whatever else you are, qualified or pre-registration, you are a learner. Though you take on multiple roles, one of them must be a learner. If you fail to attend to this aspect of your current experiences and responsibilities you may never even become a nurse or midwife. While strongly advocating a balance, the 'learner' must not be neglected. If to learn is to gain knowledge or acquire skill your role as a learner is to be actively and efficiently engaged in doing this by various methods of study, which is to apply the mind to learning. Rowntree (1998) argues that adults need to learn how to study and various strategies are introduced elsewhere in this book. Any qualified midwife or nurse will tell you how lifelong learning contributes to their professional development and how much learning they have had to undertake. It is vital therefore that you take control of the process to make it as efficient and successful as possible.

## Who is in control?

Some learners, especially if they have recently studied in a school environment, expect to be told exactly what to do, when to do it and how to do it. Their studies were closely directed and controlled by teachers. University, as you are rapidly finding out, is not like that. How difficult this may prove for a student reading history who is only required to attend the university for four hours per week! Nurses and midwives as learners face similar problems since they will have a considerable amount of time most weeks which is not timetabled. Even where it is clear what you must achieve, perhaps from explicit 'learning outcomes', the 'when' and 'how' to undertake the necessary learning will be left mainly to you.

Beliefs, whether shown to be true or false, do influence our behaviours.

- Take a glance at the sky
- What do you believe the weather will be like in two hours from now?
- How will you dress or what will you take with you assuming you must leave in fifteen minutes?

Similarly, your beliefs about your level of control will affect your activities.

## Exercise 2.1

Look at Table 2.1; on the grid where would you place yourself in terms of your own beliefs?

On this continuum of beliefs, which seeks to identify where you perceive control, it would be surprising if you selected the extreme points in relation to all of these events. It gives insight into who or what you believe is responsible for what happens to you in general. Compare your own views in a discussion with peers, family or study friends.

**Table 2.1** Control and responsibility beliefs grid

| Events/experiences | Where do you believe responsibility for these lie? |
| --- | --- |
| Acceptance on a course<br>Disappointing results in an examination<br>Experiencing good health<br>Career history | ←——————————————————————→ |

Left = Entirely outside my control and therefore not my responsibility.
Right = Entirely my own responsibility.

## Locus of control

Individuals are likely to tend towards one end of the continuum. This relates to the notion of 'locus of control', used in the psychology of health care (Surgenor *et al.*, 2000), but is equally useful in illustrating your general outlook on life and very relevant to you as a learner.

Where you sit on this continuum will influence your approach and motivation to your studies. Research suggests key differences between people who have a strong external locus of control, compared with those who have a strong internal locus of control (Gershaw, 1989). See Table 2.2.

## Are you really helpless?

There is a danger in assuming a behavioural state and mindset where a person believes they are ineffectual, their responses are futile and control over the environment is lost, described as 'learned helplessness' by Peterson *et al.* (1995), who studied this from within psychology. As with the student with a strong external locus of control, this will result in little effort or motivation to assume control over one's learning situation. While acknowledging that some things are clearly beyond our control, university education expects you to take responsibility for your own studies and there are many areas where nurses and midwives as learners must take control of themselves.

The assumption is that you value the outcome of the course or module you are studying for. It may bring better career promotion opportunities, be vital for your field of practice and, for most readers, it will secure your place on the Nursing and

**Table 2.2** Locus of control

| External | Internal |
|---|---|
| Events occur as a result of luck, fate or powerful others | Events result from one's own actions |
| The individual does not control their circumstances or the events they experience | Experiences are controlled by own skill or efforts |
| Fatalistic and passive attitude towards studies | Outcomes result from one's own actions |
| Shows little initiative | Takes responsibility as well as credit for the results of their actions |
| Limited individual responsibility | High motivation in academic performance |
| Motivation is low | |

Midwifery Council register. Your studies will make a difference to the quality of your professional practice and this is surely sufficient motive to be committed to developing study skills. An application of theory suggested by Palmgreen (1984) indicates that if

1 You value something highly (e.g. success in a difficult module) and if you believe that
2 Specific actions will produce that outcome (1), (e.g. undertaking prescribed reading and doing suggested guided-studies) then
3 The person is motivated and highly likely to engage with the specific actions (2).

Some of the exercises in this and other chapters of this book will serve to test your beliefs in this area of control and responsibility. Specific actions result in beneficial outcomes, coping and more efficient learning. You are challenged to put this to the test and you may find that taking charge can be very liberating.

## Choosing study friends

You may have no control over who you are related to but you can choose your friends. Studying can be difficult and lonely. It can feel as if you are working in the dark, uncertain if you are on track. It is worth making an effort in developing relationships with key people who have sympathy with your basic goal to succeed on your course or module.

Group work, which is set by your lecturers, will serve several purposes. But even where it is not explicitly recommended you can pool resources with study friends, meeting in rooms you can book within the university or rotating around different homes. Here you retain control and can choose to work with people from your own course or others according to factors that you have decided on.

### Study buddy

Having regular contact with one person for the purpose of encouraging mutual learning is beneficial, as common sense would tend to suggest, and this is further supported by research evidence. A study by Carr *et al.* (1996) about barriers to completing nursing or midwifery courses found that only 16% of students who did not complete the course had a study partner compared with 77% of those who did complete it. It showed that the odds of dropping out were nine times greater for a student who had no study buddy compared to students who did. Even where learning is via a virtual online environment a sense of belonging to a group is important and beneficial as Kippen (2003: 27) points out 'students who feel confident ... will congratulate each other on postings, share anecdotes, express concern if a member is "missing", and generally contribute thoughtfully to discussion'.

## Syndicate learning

This describes an organized group of individuals who meet for a specified purpose. It may be early preparation for an assignment or project and may be entirely directed by students who chose to participate. Such syndicates may be formed and disbanded according to the task requirements and can make any such work more productive than individuals working in isolation. 'TEAM', the motto proudly displayed on a grammar school notice board, stands for Together Everyone Achieves More. This maxim certainly applies to many of the learning situations that midwives, nurses and their respective students find themselves in.

## Critical friend

A study buddy may be seen more as a supportive friend and syndicate learning focuses on groups with whom you study where clear mutual benefits in your learning are obvious. Another type of relationship that is strongly advocated is someone who may be somewhat more independent of your learning situation. This person may be called upon to comment on the work you are producing and provide a 'balance between support and challenge' (Watling *et al.*, 1998:61). A 'critical friend' is a trusted person who:

- takes time to understand the context of the work
- is willing to provide an honest opinion
- asks provocative searching questions
- provides a different perspective
- offers a fairly detailed critique of a person's work
- is an advocate for the success of the work (adapted from Costa and Kallick, 1993).

Your academic supervisors will certainly fulfil some aspects of this role but it is highly recommended that you seek an independent friend to assume this role.

# Ground rules

Your university will encourage you to work closely with peers in the achievement of learning and while there may be some grey areas, which you will need to check out, working with others can be productive.

### Exercise 2.2

- Explore and locate your own university policy/guidelines on working with others
- Read this with particular attention to the concepts of cheating, collusion, plagiarism, collaboration and syndicate learning
- Any aspects which are not fully understood should become items for discussion with your personal tutor or academic supervisor
- Openly discuss these with your study friends and agree on ways of working to ensure there is no possibility of straying from these ground rules

# Emotional control

It is well recognized that both nursing and midwifery are associated with extremes of emotional situations and that learning brings its own raft of stresses and joys. Most students are concurrently engaged as learners in practice and cannot avoid the range of emotions, spanning utter despair to elation, experienced by clients and their families. Topics studied are also emotionally laden and having to study can itself become stressful. You should take control of your emotional state and acknowledge that there will be peak periods of work. A little stress can serve as a motivating force whereas too much can seriously impede your ability to think clearly or concentrate, exactly the qualities required for some aspects of effective study.

### Exercise 2.3

- Reflect on your previous life experiences, in the capacity of a learner if this is recent, and identify how you detected your emotional state
- Try to pose and answer the question 'how are you feeling?' on a regular basis
- Share these feelings with friends, study buddies, family or others you can confide in

- Adjust your own demand upon yourself if necessary
- Engage in healthy stress-relieving strategies which tend to work for you
- Seek advice, perhaps from the university student counselling service, if you go through a prolonged period where you feel limited control over your emotions

# Motivation

Your motivation may be checked at interview since it is acknowledged that to be a midwife or a nurse and study for these professions is not easy and some do not complete the course. Some candidates express vague and possibly altruistic notions of wanting to 'help people'. One student came into nursing since she had undergone life-saving surgery and wished to repay the debt she felt to the NHS. She left the course within a year, perhaps illustrating that there is a need to be realistic and clear about the demands of such a course and the profession it leads to. Clearly over a long course your motivation will fluctuate and typically somewhere around the mid-point of a course motivation will take a dip. Your personal beliefs, values and 'study friends' will help to sustain your motivation but there are things that you can do.

### Exercise 2.4

- Recall the main factors that motivated you to commence your course and what you expressed at interview
- List things which have been demotivating
- List things which still motivate you in your current studies or have revived your motivation
- Discuss these with study buddies

Things that motivate people in a learning situation include:

- being part of a group with similar experiences
- access to the resources, people or things that help coping
- developing confidence in your abilities
- gaining new knowledge which is clearly relevant
- feedback demonstrating that you have achieved something valuable.

In relation to these motivating factors, which are present in your situation and which are missing? If any appear to be missing discuss these with peers and if necessary consult your personal tutor to discuss issues.

# Goals

Having clear goals, in mind or better still written down on your personal notice board, will serve as a motivating factor. However, these may be distant and feel out of reach much of the time so it will help if you think much more in terms of short- and medium-term goals. If these are clearly leading towards your overall goal then they can be viewed as small but important steps in the right direction. Achieving your own short-term goals is rewarding and this relatively small success can be motivating.

### Exercise 2.5

- Identify a goal related to an important plan, e.g.
  - decorating your kitchen
  - obtaining part-time employment
  - a holiday in New Zealand
- List the resources you would need to make your goal feasible
- List all preparations required in advance
- What steps would you need to take as part of completing the overall goal?

Firstly it is less daunting if the goal is broken down into manageable chunks. This makes the task clearer, more feasible and shows what essential equipment, resources or skills will be required. It gives order to the overall task and suggests a starting point.

# Resources

Beware of 'dining-room table syndrome'. You will instantly recognize this if you have it! Some students, especially those who are mature in years, will live with a perpetually cluttered dining-room table which serves as makeshift 'study' for months. Romantic or even just nutritious and family-centred mealtimes become a distant memory as the course progresses. This may indicate an underlying lack of balance and control. Those in purpose-built student accommodation may have space and facilities approaching ideal but most may have to undertake some radical changes in their use of space. If you fail to control your environment it will hinder your studies. Like activities which could be described as 'preparatory', related to the 'goals' exercise above, ensuring that you have the resources for study demands an investment of time that pays dividends in terms of organizational efficiency and mental preparedness to study. The following are questions that you should have satisfactory answers to:

1   Do you have a place to study? Avoid a location that must be cleared for other purposes every day, such as kitchen surfaces or those strongly associated with distractions such as TV or sleep!
2   Is your workspace comfortable? Your seating, desk and location of your PC are important considerations if you are to avoid physical discomfort. You may need to give your space an ergonomic makeover!
3   Do you have a supply of study materials? Nice pens, highlighters, folders, post-its, A4 pad, notebook, plastic wallet files, labels, marker pens
4   Have you sufficient storage? This should allow for well-organized storage of notes etc. Clearly labelled box-files will help. Safety and moving and handling issues should be addressed, for example in the positioning of shelving
5   Have you unlimited access to computer and IT? You may need to negotiate within the family, but your needs are important. Spare consumables in stock and adequate virus-protection software. Secure devices for transporting data, e.g. project work or draft essays. Reliable broadband internet provider that is cost-effective

## Capturing time

The number of hours studying does not equate with levels of achievement, but nursing and midwifery courses come third, after medicine and veterinary science, in the number of study hours required to obtain a degree (Bekhradnia *et al.*, 2006:6). It has been pointed out that the amount of time is not the issue. It is how time is utilized that is important (Northedge, 2005:34). Nevertheless you must capture sufficient time each week and protect it for efficient use. Like income, there are amounts that are pre-allocated, for fees, food and fashions, and hopefully some spare to dispose of as you wish. Initially you will need to take stock to establish what you actually spend, invest or squander your time on.

### Exercise 2.6

• List things which you do regularly and allocate an approximate weekly amount of hours, devoted to each activity. Ensure you overestimate rather than underestimate these amounts. The following categories may prevent important omissions:

- ○ sleep
- ○ hygiene
- ○ travel
- ○ course attendance
- ○ shopping
- ○ preparation of meals and eating
- ○ employment
- ○ relaxation
- ○ responsibilities
- ○ regular commitments
- Base this exercise on a typical week, preferably one since the course commenced
- Calculate the weekly total and subtract this figure from 168, the number of hours in seven days. This gives you an estimate of the spare time you have control over – 'disposable' time
- Consider how this must be altered when you are on placements, if applicable


# The three D's

It is likely that you have identified a number of 'disposable' hours, which must now be carefully invested. If you are left wondering where all your apparently 'spare time' goes you may need to extend your analysis by logging the actual use made of your time by drawing up and completing a grid over one whole week. If you are typical, there may be an astonishingly large amount of time devoted to watching television! You may need to release time and allocate your disposable time according to your individual priorities and here the three D's can be very useful.

**Delegate** There may be regular commitments or responsibilities which eat into time required for your studies. Yet these things need doing and you should use the support of family and friends to delegate some of these. I usually suggest that teenagers within the family are given a crash course in ironing and other housework tasks!

**Defer** Certain of your regular commitments, social aspirations or pleasures may have to be placed on hold and deferred until holiday periods, times where study is less intensive or even beyond the course completion. The use of DVDs to store up 'must-see' television and other deferred pleasures can be used as incentives to complete coursework. These become personal rewards for achievement of your medium-term goals.

**Delete** In the light of the value you place on success in your course there will be a price to pay. Commitment is required and you must set realistic priorities. This will mean that to free up disposable time to invest in the course some tasks or regular commitments may have to simply be deleted.

In spite of this, maintaining a balance is important. Some things must be retained. In planning this investment you should be realistic and ensure that one day is completely free from study. The defence that you simply have not got enough time is attractive but reflects a defeatist attitude something like the anonymous piece in Table 2.3.

However, the real issue is how to control and utilize the hours that are available.

**Table 2.3** Days in a year!

| Days left | There are 365 days in a year! | Days |
| --- | --- | --- |
| 365 | Minus Sundays the day of rest | 52 |
| 313 | Minus summer holidays when it is too hot to study | 50 |
| 263 | Eight hours sleep per night | 130 |
| 141 | One hour a day for playing which is good for health | 15 |
| 126 | Two hours daily for food intake | 30 |
| 96 | One hour a day for talking as man is a social being | 15 |
| 81 | Exam days | 35 |
| 46 | Bank holidays | 40 |
| 6 | Sickness | 3 |
| 3 | Going to the movies and days out | 2 |
| 1 | You cannot work on your birthday! | 1 |
| 0 | Days left for studying! | 0 |

# Taking control of your timetable

Set a realistic timetable and review achievements each week. It is worthwhile using a template and having a paper copy on display such as the example in Table 2.4. You may simply use a planner found in many software packages and you may wish to be more detailed, but do remain realistic and ensure you accommodate important activities you identified in the previous exercise.

**Table 2.4** Weekly study timetable

|  | Morning | Afternoon | Evening |
|---|---|---|---|
| **Monday** | Lectures | Squash + library | Sociology essay |
| **Tuesday** | Read Chapter 8 | Lectures | Meet and eat with syndicate group |
| **Wednesday** | Lie in + reflective diary + prep for tutorial on Friday | Placement | |
| **Thursday** | Placement | | Revise stages of labour, physiology and complications |
| **Friday** | Lectures + tutorial | Prepare for ethics seminar due next week | Evening off |
| **Saturday** | Home – job list e.g. fix bike | Catch-up study session | Review week – timetable (1 hour only) Meet friends |
| **Sunday** | Family – NO STUDY TODAY | | |

'Parkinsons' Law', of no connection with the common neurological disease, states that 'work expands to fill up the time available'. If you have three months to complete an essay, it will take three months at least, but if it must be submitted in three weeks from today, you *could* manage to meet that deadline. Therefore being generous in allocating time to tasks may not represent its most efficient use.

Guidelines for developing a realistic weekly timetable:

- Refer to your course plan showing key deadline dates
- Consult your social calendar and ensure time is allocated, e.g. 'nephew's wedding'
- Make sure pleasurable social events are seen as legitimate, e.g. squash
- Allocate tougher tasks to timeslots when you are generally best able to concentrate, e.g. between 7.30 and 10pm, or before 11am
- Allocate 'catch-up' time to accommodate inevitable slippage

- Take account of your review of the previous week in devising next week's timetable
- Allocated study time should be subject to more detailed planning and ensure that each time slot has a written specific purpose

### Lessons from a coach driver

This true story was related on a radio programme some years ago and shows a mindset which takes control of time. The coach was being driven empty on the return to the depot and became stuck in motorway traffic. Time passed with no sign of movement so, checking regularly from his vantage point, the driver picked up the litter left by his passengers. He then cleaned all of the internal windows. Still in stationary traffic he got off, collected his step-ladder and proceeded to wash the external windows. On completion there were signs of movement as he stowed the equipment and took his seat. Time was invested rather than spent. The point here is a readiness to capture even short time slots that become available and this may require carrying your notebook and current shopping list of study tasks.

### Exercise 2.7

- Consider this list of possible study activities you will need to be engaged with
  - critical reading of a complex article
  - discussion with peers
  - gathering information for a seminar
  - memorizing a physiological sequence
  - planning for future deadlines
  - project work with others
  - redrafting an essay
  - reflection on an incident in practice
  - revision for an assessment
- Add anything which has been omitted
- Categorize these activities on the following two dimensions
  - needs relatively small amount of time – needs a substantial time slot
  - can be achieved with little concentration – needs clear thinking and undisturbed concentration

It may become clear that while some activities require intense concentration or prolonged time slots, others can be interrupted without harm and be achieved in quite small amounts of time, i.e. just 15 or 30 minutes.

You may come across the idea of learning being either 'deep' or 'surface'. Deep learning occurs when students approach a task with the goal of understanding it as well as possible. Learning will be surface when students approach a task with a goal of getting an overview or completing it as quickly as possible, often to simply meet assessment requirements (Evans & Abbot, 1998). Surface and deep approaches to learning are not personality traits, but can represent the strategy you choose to employ in different learning situations. So you control the approach you take. Glancing back at the list of activities above you may be able to match the approach to the task in hand.

# Conclusions

This chapter has directed you to look at yourself, examine your beliefs about being a learner and has challenged you take more responsibility for your learning. This has involved taking control of your time and prioritizing its use. It has mainly tried to get you to consider not how intelligent or gifted you are but how organized and 'smart' you are in taking control of yourself as a learner. *SMART learners will display many of the following characteristics:*

S  – Strategic
M – Motivated
A  – Analytical and Active
R  – Realistic, Resourceful and Responsible
T  – Takes control of own learning and Time

As you become more SMART as a learner you can be pleased to know that within the time you have captured you are focused on effective activities and equipped to assume more control and credit for your small achievements and long-term success as a learner.

# 3

# Making information work for nursing and midwifery students

*Introduction • Information technology • Library • Library layout • Book arrangements • Journal arrangements • Library networks • Passwords • Reading lists and references • Catalogue • Sources of information • Journals • Official publications • Databases • Search engines • Websites • Core websites • Handling, presenting and storing information • Handling information • File management and data storage • Viruses, worms and spyware • Conclusions*

Information can be defined as any idea, concept, fact, opinion or knowledge that can be communicated. This chapter will help you understand the role that information will play in your studies, the way it is stored and the ways in which you can find it. It covers information technology and efficient use of the library which is vital in relation to the reading lists and references you will receive. The following are also given attention: searching the library catalogue, sources of information, useful databases and how to assess the quality of websites. Much of the information you need will be in electronic format making handling, presenting, storing information, file management and avoiding viruses important skills. Collectively these topics will help you to make information work for you.

# Introduction

> Research means that you don't know, but are willing to find out.
>
> Charles F. Kettering

Some information you will already have, that which has come from your experience. Some information you will get by observing, practising, reading or reflecting on your activities. Clearly the qualified nurse or midwife will have a lot more professional experience than a novice student but you will be surprised how life experiences provide much relevant information.

A professional practitioner in the course of their work should be able to look at a problem, find possible answers, develop a way of dealing with the problem and check that it works. You may be asked by a patient for a drink of water so you will need to check that the patient is allowed a drink, and then you will need to find a glass and a source of drinking water. Qualified nurses and midwives will be constantly identifying problems, finding and applying solutions and checking the results without even stopping to think about them.

As a student you will be asked to write essays and many other types of written assignments for your learning to be assessed. In the course of preparing and writing an assignment you will need to be able to identify questions, find and assess information to answer them and check that what you have written answers the question. Finding information to write an essay mirrors the problem-solving skills you will need to develop as a competent practitioner.

So the ability to find and use information will be an important part of your role both as a professional nurse or midwife and as a student studying those subjects. The library will play a central role in your studies at university, so investing time in learning how to use the library and its resources will be repaid in time saved. We do not normally think about how we use information until we begin studying and need to find things in the library and to use computers to find things on the Internet. Research undertaken by Shorten and Wallace (2001) has shown that students who spend time gaining information literacy skills have improved levels of self-confidence in their academic writing abilities.

# Information technology

Few people these days do not know what computers are used for in the home. They can be used for games, booking holidays, writing essays, storing photographs, downloading music and finding information. The ability to use a computer when you begin to study enables you to: find information, write essays, keep a log of your experience and most importantly save time.

You will also need to be able to use computers confidently when you become qualified nurses or midwives. The NHS has invested many millions of pounds in computer systems to decrease the amount of paperwork in circulation and reduce the time a patient has to wait. In the future much of this work will be undertaken using the NHS computer network. The following systems are currently being developed:

- **Choose and book** – will allow patients to choose the date and time of appointments
- **NHS care records** – electronic patient records, accessible to patients and carers
- **Electronic transmission of prescriptions (ETP)** – electronic prescription forms
- **NHS mail** – an email service for all NHS employees
- **Picture archiving and communications systems (PACS)** – electronic transfer of images, scans and x-rays
- **Expert patient online** – online training for patients with long-term conditions.

People are becoming increasingly interested in their own health and turn to the Internet for information on health problems. Health advice, patient support and information on specific disorders such as cancer and heart disease can be readily found on the Internet.

A Harris Online poll found that patients who use the Internet to look for health information are more likely to ask more specific and informed questions of their doctors and to comply with prescribed treatment plans (Anon 2001).

With the development of knowledgeable patients, nurses and midwives have to be very well informed in order to answer questions and reassure patients about their condition and possible treatment regimes.

# Library

Your university library should be the first place to visit when you are looking for information. The size of a university library may appear daunting to students who are used to their school or public libraries but it is reassuring to know that libraries whether they are tiny or huge are all organized in a similar way. Most universities allow new students the opportunity of taking a tour of the library during Freshers' or Induction Week to introduce them to their librarian and to show them where the books for their course are. If you have not been provided with a tour you can always ask at a library enquiry desk and they will usually organize a brief tour. You can also pick up guides and other printed material from your library, which explains what resources are available and how to use them. University libraries come in all sorts of shapes and sizes. They can be in a single block with different subjects on each floor or there may be a smaller nursing and midwifery library attached to a health studies department or a hospital trust.

The subject librarian will have consulted with the nursing and midwifery lecturers to decide on the specific books and other resources you will need to refer to on your course. Many of the resources will be available over the Internet so you will be able to work from home or even from your practice placement.

It is always a good idea to get to know the subject librarian who looks after nursing and midwifery. The subject librarian will have responsibility for buying books and journals to support the nursing and midwifery modules. Most subject librarians will also spend a lot of time helping students to study by teaching them how to use the library and its resources. So do not hesitate to contact the librarian if you are at all concerned about using the library.

## Library layout

Each library will look different but will essentially contain the same things. There will be books and journals (magazines), student computers, study areas, printers, photocopiers and enquiry desks.

## Book arrangements

Books in academic libraries are usually put on the library shelves in subject order. This is to enable you to find all the books on a particular subject. To do this subject librarians look at the book, decide what subject or subjects it contains and give it a code. The code is taken from a classification scheme: the two most commonly used in academic libraries are Dewey Decimal Classification (DDC) and Library of Congress (LOC), but there are others. If you look at the spine of a book in the library you will see a label with either numbers or letters or a combination of both. These are called the class mark, shelf mark or call number. The call number tells you where to find a book on the shelves but you will also learn that each number will tell you what the book is about. Table 3.1 illustrates the codes allocated for different aspects of medicine.

The following book reference could have either of the codes in bold depending on the classification used in your library.

Hinchliff, S. (2003) Nursing practice and healthcare. London: Arnold

DDC Number **610.73 NUR**

LOC Number **RT42. N868 2003**

**Table 3.1** Library classification schemes

| Dewey Decimal (DDC) | | Library of Congress | |
|---|---|---|---|
| Code | Subject | Code | Subject |
| 610 | Medical sciences | R | Medicine |
| 611 | Human anatomy | RB | Pathology |
| 612 | Human physiology | RC | Internal medicine |
| 613 | Health promotion | RG | Gynecology/obstetrics |
| 614 | Public health | RJ | Pediatrics |
| 615 | Therapeutics | RK | Dentistry |
| 616 | Diseases, surgery | RM | Pharmacology |
| 617 | Gynaecology/obstetrics | RT | Nursing |
| 618 | Paediatrics, geriatrics | RV–RZ | Alternative medicine |

# Journal arrangements

In addition to books you will learn to use journals. Journals can also be called serials, periodicals or magazines. Journals are used a lot because they contain specific up-to-date information. Printed journals, unlike books, are filed in alphabetical order by the title. They are normally stored separately from the books and may even be on a different floor of the library.

# Library networks

All libraries are part of a network so in addition to your university library you may be able to use the libraries based at the NHS trusts where you undertake your practice placements. The NHS libraries normally have agreements with the local university to provide students with services. Qualified nurses and midwives undertaking courses will, as employees, be entitled to NHS library membership. You will need to check with your university library exactly what you can expect while you are on placement. Students on placement can normally expect support from their library in the form of access to other libraries, online resources, extended or postal loans and online consultation services.

There are other organizations such as the Royal College of Nursing (RCN) and Royal College of Midwives (RCM) who offer library services to nurses and midwives. Student nurses and midwives in addition to qualified staff can become members.

# Passwords

While people are familiar with PIN numbers and passwords in everyday life most are less familiar with the concept of passwords to use resources. There are a range of usernames and passwords that students have to become familiar with, in order to make best use of all of the university's resources. You will be told how to obtain your passwords during your induction week. Many universities now use a portal that requires a single password to gain access to all library resources. Even if you prefer to work from home you may be required to use a range of passwords.

Depending on your university you may need to make use of all of these passwords:

- **Athens** – a password system that allows access to a range of online resources including databases, ejournals and ebooks
- **Network** – a password that allows access to the university computer network
- **Online Learning Environment** – a password that allows access to WebCT, Blackboard or any other online learning environment
- **Portal** – a password that allows access to online resources
- **Individual** – a few resources require individual passwords.

# Reading lists and references

During your studies you may be given a reading list. This is a list of references to book titles, journal articles and other publications your lecturer advises you to read. Normally a list is divided into *essential* and *recommended* reading. Usually you do not have to read everything on the list but you should read at least one of the essential readings and a selection of the recommended references. Your library should contain copies of the titles on the reading list. Increasingly however, references will be to online publications such as websites, reports and journals that can be found by typing the universal resource locator (URL) http://www.document.ac.uk, into your web browser. See Table 3.2 and Figures 3.1 and 3.2.

**Table 3.2** Examples of reading list references

| Format | Example |
| --- | --- |
| Book | Basford, L., Slevin, O. (eds) (2001) *Theory and Practice of Nursing: An Integrated Approach to Patient Care.* 2nd ed. Cheltenham, Nelson Thornes |
| Journal article | Waine, W., Scullion, P. (2002) A new model for the nursing research agenda. *Nursing Management* 9(2): 18–23 |
| Official publication | World Health Organization, UNICEF (1978) Primary Health Care: Joint Report (by the Director-General of the World Health Organization and the Executive Director of the United Nations Children's Fund). Geneva: WHO |
| Online publication | Great Britain, Department of Health (2004) *Choosing Health – Making healthy choices easier.* [online] London, Stationery Office. Available from http://www.dh.gov.uk/assetRoot/04/12/07/92/04120792.pdf (19th April 2006) |

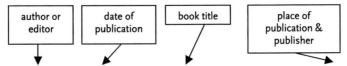

Hinchliff, S. (2003) *Nursing practice and health care.* London: Arnold

**FIGURE 3.1** Elements of a book reference

# Catalogue

The online catalogue or OPAC (Online Public Access Catalogue) is used to find books, journals and other resources in the library. Whether you are familiar with computers or not, the catalogue is very easy to use. To find the information you

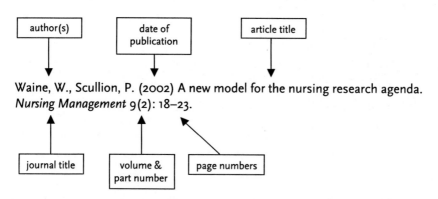

FIGURE 3.2  Elements of a journal article reference

will require quickly, knowing how to use the catalogue is an essential skill. The general rule to remember is, the less you type the more you find. Make sure that you have not mistyped or misspelt the information you type in and always double check.

### Searching the catalogue

You can search the catalogue in many different ways. Table 3.3 explains what each search looks for. The keyword and the author/title searches are used to quickly find resources while more specific searches can be employed to find particular resources. If you learn to use the catalogue it will pay dividends in the time you will save looking for items in the library.

**Table 3.3** Library catalogue search terms

| Search by | What it will look for |
| --- | --- |
| Keyword | Word or words anywhere in the record |
| Keyword title | Word or words that appear in the title |
| Author/title | Any combination of surname and keyword |
| Subject heading | Subject content |
| Author | Author's surname and initial |
| Class/shelf mark | Subject code allocated to the title |
| ISBN | International Standard Book Number |
| Journal title | Words in journal title |

For example:

- If you are looking for a book on 'study skills for nurses and midwives' you could type 'study skills nurses' or 'study skills midwives' and you would find everything in the library with that combination of words in the title
- If you are looking for a particular book such as 'Norman, I. and Ryrie, I. (2004) *The Art and Science of Mental Health Nursing*. Maidenhead, Open University' you could type 'Norman Mental' or 'Norman Health' and you would find all the titles in the library written by Norman with the words mental or health in the title

# Sources of information

In a library information comes packaged in lots of different formats. Everyone has used a book at some point in their studies, but less common, yet of great importance, are reports, journals and official publications. In your studies you may need to thoroughly investigate a topic, so it is worth getting to know the different formats in which information is packaged, when to use them, and how to assess their value.

Books, journals and official publications are called primary sources because they contain information you can use directly. Secondary sources are normally used to locate primary sources. Secondary sources include bibliographies, databases, search engines and websites.

## Books

Books come in two distinct types. Textbooks that give an overview of a subject may be specially written to support a branch of study or a particular course. They are usually quite large, with lots of illustrations or diagrams and have lots of headings and subheadings. The other type, called monographs, are scholarly books written on a specific aspect of, or approach to, a subject. So you could find a textbook on nursing practice but you would find a monograph on heart disease in the elderly or episiotomy in midwifery practice. Increasingly core textbooks are being published in both print and online versions so it will be worth checking which online textbooks are available to you.

## Book assessment criteria

In your first year, books should form the basis of your information gathering but you should not rely on them for all of your information needs. You should also be able to assess the quality of a book before you use it. See Table 3.4.

**Table 3.4** Book assessment criteria

| Criteria | What to look for |
|---|---|
| Date of publication | How old is it? Have things changed? Are there newer editions? |
| Author or editor | What experience or qualifications do they have? |
| Style | Contents page and index? Informal or academic? Easy to read? |
| Publisher | Academic? Government, profession or pressure group? |
| Edition | The latest edition will contain the most up-to-date information |

TIP: Have a look at some of the books on any of the reading lists your tutor gives you as this will give you an idea of the types of books you need to use.

# Journals

Journals, magazines, periodicals or serials: all these names relate to publications that are published in parts over a period of time. They can be published in both print and electronic formats and arrive in the library weekly, monthly, quarterly or six-monthly. Journal articles will become a significant source of information in your studies because it is where the majority of recent research-based information is published.

Although there are a wide range of journal titles covering all aspects of nursing and midwifery, the articles within them are normally found using an electronic database or index. Increasingly journals are being published in an electronic form that allows you to use your computer to find the information you need, download the article and then print it out. However, it is worth remembering that older articles will come from print journals and not all of the newer journals will be available on the Internet and even when they are there could be a fee to pay. It is important to check what journals your library takes to support your specific course. To do this you will have to use the catalogue, portal or ask at the library enquiry desk.

# Official publications

During your studies you will need information about government legislation, health service policy and the regulations that govern nursing and midwifery. These are called official publications, and include anything published by the Government such as Acts of Parliament, Green Papers, White Papers and official reports. You could also include publications by the Department of Health, Stationery Office, Nursing and Midwifery Council (NMC) and the Royal Colleges. An aim of the Government is to make information available and many official publications can now be downloaded from the Internet. For those working in the National Health Service, the Department of Health website has a database containing a range of online documents relating to the NHS. There is a website with the full text of all Acts of Parliament published since 1996 (http://www.opsi.gov.uk/legislation/about_legislation.htm). Older printed Acts of Parliament will normally be kept in your library and can be found using the catalogue. However, it is often easy to use the simplified guides to relevant acts rather than the actual acts which are written in legal language that may be inaccessible to the average nursing or midwifery student. A good example is Blackstone's guide to the Mental Capacity Act 2005 (Bartlett, 2005) which forms part of a series of guides to important Acts. See Table 3.5.

**Table 3.5** Types of government publication

| Type of publication | What they mean |
| --- | --- |
| Act of Parliament | A law or piece of legislation enacted by Parliament |
| Parliamentary Bill | A draft Act presented to Parliament |
| White Paper | Statement of government policy or proposed legislation |
| Green Paper | A discussion document of proposed legislation |
| Statutory instrument | Secondary legislation not needing parliamentary assent |
| Parliamentary Papers | Publications made at the request of Parliament |
| Non-Parliamentary Papers | Publications from government departments |

Other semi-official organizations publish a range of documents both in print and online, which you may need to use. The NMC publishes guidance for students and qualified nurses and midwives. The Royal Colleges also have a range of documentation and services to support student and qualified staff in their education.

# Databases

A database is an electronic index that allows you to locate information in journals without searching individual issues. Most databases allow you to search by subject, keyword, journal title or author of the article. A database uses human expertise to assess the quality and accuracy of the information.

They also index to a set of headings that illustrate the subject content of journal articles, case studies, clinical trials, dissertations, practice guidelines and systematic reviews.

Databases normally come in two types: bibliographic and full text. Full text databases are usually less comprehensive than bibliographic ones but you will be able to download articles directly. Bibliographic databases contain only references to information but there are often links to local journal holdings both in print and electronic. They contain more subject-specific information and have many more references. Usually there are tools in a bibliographic database that let you focus your search, manipulate your search results and, very usefully, save them to disk or email a list of references to yourself. See Table 3.6.

**Table 3.6** Main health databases

| Database | Subjects covered |
| --- | --- |
| Amed | Complementary medicine, allied health, palliative care |
| ASSIA | Social issues, social problems, health, gender and ethnicity issues |
| CINAHL | All aspects of allied health, nursing and midwifery |
| Medline | Medicine, nursing, midwifery, surgery and rehabilitation |
| NMI | UK biased index of nursing and midwifery journal literature |
| PsycINFO | All aspects of general and clinical psychology |
| Pubmed | Medicine, nursing, midwifery, surgery and rehabilitation |

# Search engines

Search engines such as AltaVista, Google and Ask are the tools most of us use to search the Internet. They search the Internet for keywords or images found in websites. Whereas a database uses human expertise to index the entries a search engine indexes the content automatically. So the accuracy and quality of the information found by the search engine will not be assessed. It is worth remembering that search engines are commercial organizations that charge companies to promote websites.

Search engines are an easy-to-use tool for finding information for nurses and midwives but the information they find needs to be treated with caution. In general a search engine is good for finding documents such as the NMC Code of Conduct (2004), patient information or by using the Image Search option, an illustration of the human lungs, but less accurate for clinical information. See Table 3.7.

**Table 3.7** Search engine searching tips

| Tool | What does it do? |
| --- | --- |
| Speech marks '' | 'National Service Frameworks' will find the phrase |
| Plus sign + | Using the + sign means the word must be found |
| Minus sign − | Using the − sign means the word should not be found |
| Advanced search | Complicated searches using a search form format |

There are a number of tools that you can use that will help to simplify your searches.

### Intute: health and life sciences – nursing, midwifery and allied health

Intute is a search engine supported by a number of higher education institutes. It is subject-based and searches for relevant websites from an indexed database. The content of the database is selected and quality assessed by a panel of subject experts, who also add subject terms for easier searching. It also includes an online internet search tutorial specially designed for nursing and midwifery students to develop the skills needed to be able to quality assess websites for themselves.

### Google Scholar

If you are looking for clinical information and you do not have access to a database you can use Google Scholar which will search for peer-reviewed academic papers. As with a database you can search by author, article title, keyword or source. It will link directly to the article or to the abstract. You can also look at references that have cited the articles you have found. It also has an advanced search facility that will allow you to make more detailed searches. However, if you do have access to commercial databases then use them or Intute in preference, as their content will not need quality assessing.

# Websites

Most organizations have a website to promote their products, support their ideals and sustain their members. Some websites have an area that can be accessed only if you are a member of the organization, whilst others allow the public to freely access information and publications. Websites are a useful source of information but care should be taken that they are used in conjunction with other information sources.

### Website assessment criteria

When using websites care has to be taken that they supply unbiased, accurate and up-to-date information. Table 3.8 will help you assess if a website meets those criteria.

**Table 3.8** Website assessment criteria

| Criteria | What to look for |
| --- | --- |
| Authority | Are the author's/sponsor's qualifications available? |
| | Do they have expertise in this subject? |
| | Is the author/sponsor connected to an educational institution or other reputable organization? |
| | Is contact information for the author/sponsor available on the site? |
| Coverage | Is the information on the site relevant to your topic? |
| | Do you think it will be useful to you? |
| | Does this page have information that is not found elsewhere? |
| | How in-depth is the material? |
| Currency | When was the site last updated? (check the bottom of the web page) |
| | Check the information on the page and compare it to other sources |
| | Do all of the links on the site work? |
| Objectivity | Does the site display any form of bias? |
| | Does the page present facts and not try to sway opinion? |
| | Is the page free of advertisements or sponsored links? |
| Usability | Does the page look cluttered? |
| | Is it easy to find what you are looking for? |
| | Is there a menu or guide? |
| | Do you need to download additional software? |

TIP: Have a look at some of the websites your lecturer recommends. This will give you an idea of a good website.

# Core websites

### Exercise 3.1

There are a number of core websites that nursing and midwifery students should be using regularly. You may find links to them on the university web pages, electronic learning environment or the student portal but it is still worthwhile learning how to find them on the Internet. Click onto http://www.intute.ac.uk and see if you can find the following websites:

- Department of Health – see if you can find the publications library
- Nursing and Midwifery Council – see if you can find the Code of Conduct
- Royal College of Nursing – have a look at the latest news
- Royal College of Midwives – have a look at the student services page.

TIP: If you learn to navigate around core websites you will save time.


# Handling, presenting and storing information

When you have gathered the information you require from the library and other sources you will need to put it into a format that can be read, saved or presented. Most universities prefer assignments to be in an electronic format, therefore typing becomes an essential skill to acquire; in addition familiarity with the relevant software packages will pay dividends in time saved and stress avoided. Microsoft Office© is the most commonly used suite of programs used to handle information in both printed and electronic formats. It comprises the following individual programs:

- Microsoft Word© is a word processing program for creating documents of all types including web pages. You can create, format, edit, insert tables, pictures, symbols into documents and save onto disk, CD or memory stick
- Microsoft PowerPoint© is a program designed to produce presentations which can be printed as a handout or projected as slides onto a screen. You can insert graphics, special effects, graphs and tabular information into the slides to present your ideas or findings
- Microsoft Excel© is a program designed to calculate numerical data and present it in tables, graphs, PIE or bar charts
- Microsoft Internet Explorer© is the most commonly used web browser. A web browser communicates with the Internet and allows you to search for web pages and save them for later use
- Microsoft Outlook© is a communications and personal management program that allows you to send and receive emails, set up timetables and arrange appointments
- Microsoft Access© is a database program that allows you to store data such as addresses or references.

Many students, nurses and midwives will be familiar with most of these programs as they are so widely used in most large organizations such as the NHS and higher education. However, there are alternatives that you may be familiar with such as Microsoft Works© or Wordperfect©.

# Handling information

### Exercise 3.2

If you are unfamiliar with word processing or any other software there are a number of online instruction tutorials available on the Internet. Click onto www.google.com and see if you can find tutorials to help you learn.

- Type: 'Typing Tutorial' and pick one that suits you
- Type: +Microsoft +Word +Tutorial and pick one that suits you
- Type: +Microsoft +PowerPoint +Tutorial and pick one that suits you

# File management and data storage

When you have typed your assignment you will need to save it somewhere. There are a number of alternatives:

- Floppy Disk (A: drive) – low capacity portable disk
- Hard Disk (C: drive) – very high capacity disk integral to your PC
- Remote Drive (P: drive) – high capacity disk built into a university PC network
- CD or DVD (D: drive) – high capacity portable disk needing special software
- Memory Stick (E: drive) – high capacity plug-in device.

Different types of file will have different endings or extensions:

- yourassignment.doc – this will be a Word document
- yourassignment.txt – this will be a plain text file
- yourassignment.html – this will be a web page
- yourassignment.ppt – this will be a PowerPoint presentation.

The computer will give the file an address where it can be found. See Figure 3.3.

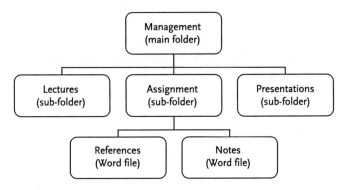

**FIGURE 3.3**  File management

## Exercise 3.3

Look at the following file addresses and see if you can work out where the files are on the above diagram, what drive they are on, and the type of file they are.

- A:/management/lectures/notes.doc
- C:/management/assignment/references/module.txt
- P:/management/presentations/overview.ppt

# Viruses, worms and spyware

Although most university computer networks are well protected by antivirus software many home computers and laptops are not. It may be a setback to lose an essay or project but it will be a disaster if your bank account is emptied or your identity is stolen. Remember the more unknown disks you allow into your computer slot the higher the chance of contracting a virus.

# Conclusions

The title of this chapter is 'Making information work for you' which sums up what you need to be able to do. You need to make the information provided by lecturers, practitioners and the library work to make you a competent practitioner. Libraries have been around since the time of the pyramids, collecting and storing information. During that time they have developed structured systematic ways of finding the information that they store. If you invest some time in learning how a library and its resources work it will be repaid in triplicate later in your studies.

What should you remember?

- That information comes in lots of formats provided by the library and people you meet
- That information to support your learning will be available but you will need to spend some time to find it
- That not all information is suitable for use in an assignment and you will need to assess its quality before you use it
- Not to rely on the Internet for all your information as it may lead to poor results in assessments
- Make contact with your subject librarian who will be an invaluable friend to both help you find information and to teach you how to use valuable resources.

In Chapter 6 we learn how to undertake the scientific process of a literature search. This chapter will look in detail at defining and refining search terms in order that a comprehensive search of the scientific literature can be completed.

# Part 2

## Beginning to develop effective study skills

# 4

# Strategies for successful learning in nursing and midwifery

*Introduction • Learning • Learning as an active process • Disability and learning • Reading • Mind maps • Writing an essay • Conclusion*

The desirable end results of your study efforts is that learning occurs, and so this chapter commences with a brief introduction to concepts related to learning. Valuable learning takes place within clinical practice, often using reflection as the key strategy. As this is of such importance it is covered separately in Chapter 5. Students experience numerous learning difficulties, such as dyslexia, many of which are fully compatible with the demands of the university and professional roles. Advice is offered to those who may experience such difficulties. The emphasis here is on university-based learning concentrating on strategies for effective reading, note taking and the use of mind maps. Learning must be communicated and you will frequently be expected to produce essays, a demand which gives rise to some common anxieties. Therefore strategies for effective essay writing are given detailed consideration in this chapter including 'task analysis' and how to check your essay drafts.

# Introduction

You may have been studying for years and feel that your results show that you are a successful learner. For many people studying does not appear to come naturally and even if you have a commendable track record of success, the demands of a nursing or midwifery course at university will be different and your learning strategies may not be as efficient as they could be. Rowntree (1998:2), from his wealth of experience and research with university students, points out starkly that in order to keep up-to-date and maintain our employability most people 'are going to be studying, off and on, formally or informally, throughout our working years, if not beyond'. This certainly applies to adult learners in nursing and midwifery who need to learn how to study.

All of the strategies outlined require active participation and motivation driven by your own priorities. But they provide ideas, structures and tools for successful learning in nursing and midwifery.

# Learning

Learning is often conceptualized as a change in behaviour, attitudes or knowledge which is relatively permanent and results from experiences rather than simply physiological maturation. These experiences may be deliberate or totally unplanned.

Passive learning occurs as a result of exposure to events and may happen simply as a result of being in a particular environment. If you work in a shop, even without effort, you will pick up things about this sector concerning customer relations, health and safety and stock control. Similarly you will learn the unwritten rules and the accepted norms of nursing or midwifery by being immersed in the culture, both in the university and practice settings. This explains, in part, the socialization processes which result in novice midwifery and nursing students becoming professional people.

'Study', however, is an active and deliberate activity and this may be seen as the process while 'learning' is often conceived of as the outcome.

Figure 4.1 shows a simplified model of learning which illustrates the link between experience and behaviour. Experiences that result in learning are of course endless but pertinent examples include:

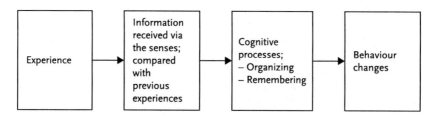

FIGURE 4.1  Link between experience and behaviour

- watching television news or documentaries
- discussions with a client or relative
- attending a lecture, seminar or involvement in 'role-play' activity
- deliberately thinking or reflecting
- online discussion with a physiotherapy student
- reading textbooks, articles or web pages etc.

Our behaviour may demonstrate that learning has occurred in many ways such as:

- explaining something clearly to somebody else
- performance in a test or quiz
- carrying out a practical procedure such as taking physiological measurements
- displaying a positive attitude, e.g. respect to a client who is refusing treatment
- writing an essay which demonstrates understanding or higher-level skills.

# Learning as an active process

The process of learning is enhanced in terms of understanding and remembering when it is made an active process. It has been found that students who actively engage with the material are more likely to recall information and will therefore be able to use it in different contexts (Bruner, 1961). Robins and Mayer (1993) argue that learning depends on cognitive activity and you are strongly advised to ensure that your learning experiences and deliberate study are not passive.

The single most important factor in preventing forgetting and enhancing longer-term memory is to review key ideas at the end of a teaching session (Cooperstein and Kocevar-Weidinger, 2004). This is because the greatest reduction in memory occurs immediately after the learning experience, making this review and then periodic recall of material important strategies to enhance memory.

These ideas have general application but in this context you can study actively by LEARN.

- Look – listen – do; using more than one of your senses; if you can hear, see and do a learning activity this is better than simply listening
- Employ a reading strategy
- Aids to memory, such as the use of mnemonics (LEARN) or visual images
- Review frequently; timetable short periods to review learning
- Notes, written in your own words.

# Disability and learning

Disabled people are by no means barred from nursing or midwifery. There are health professionals with hearing impairments, epilepsy, diabetes and depression. Such people may adopt effective strategies to enable them to learn which may be peculiar to their own circumstances. A qualified health professional may negotiate out of an internal shift rotation system if this seriously disrupts the control of their diabetes or epilepsy related to diet or medication. There are courses in mental health nursing which are taught bilingually for Deaf students and hearing students together using British Sign Language and spoken English. Resources designed to support healthcare professionals and students who happen to also be disabled people are available (Wright, 1999). Many disabled people have had successful careers in nursing and midwifery based on successful learning and some have become disability champions within the NHS (Anon, 2004).

While many people are familiar with their own impairments, indeed they become experts about themselves, quite a number of nursing and midwifery students discover they have a learning disability after commencing their course. Ideally if you are aware or suspect you may have a recognized learning difficulty such as dyslexia you should take advice in advance of commencing your course. Your university disabilities officer will provide initial advice that will often include how to obtain an assessment. After a formal assessment you may be eligible for Disabled Students Allowance (Scottish Executive, 2006) which is a financial benefit designed to cover certain extra expenses which arise because you are on a course. All nursing and midwifery students, whether in receipt of an NHS bursary or not, are able to apply for Disabled Students Allowance which may fund a dyslexia support tutor or specialist software.

Organizations providing employment or educational services have a legal obligation to make necessary reasonable adjustments for employees or students who are 'disabled' according to the legal definition, which is surprisingly broad. What you can expect from the university and its associated clinical placement providers will depend on your specific circumstances. The 'reasonable adjustments' made will not mean that standards are lowered but may include the provision of:

- specialized software which assists in note taking and spell checking
- longer loan periods for items and access to specialized reading equipment in the library
- a person to take notes for you in lectures
- additional time in exam situations
- support in the preparation of essays, e.g. a proofreading service
- permission to make an audio recording of lectures
- provision of notes (handouts) from the lecturer on coloured paper if necessary.

In assessments the standards remain unaltered but the reasonable adjustments are made to assist students with a recognized learning difficulty in achieving these standards.

# Reading

When you go to university you are said to be reading for a degree. However, even if you are undertaking a diploma or short CPD course, reading will nevertheless take up a lot of your available study time. It is worth spending some time learning how to make reading active and efficient so that you can spend more time on other important things.

## Parts of a book

Most strategies for reading efficiently and effectively apply equally irrespective of the type of material you are reading: book, journal article, report or web pages. As books form a large proportion of the materials you must use, familiarizing yourself with the structure of a book is worthwhile. Academic books come in two broad categories: monographs which are books on a specific subject and textbooks which contain information to support a branch of study. Textbooks and monographs will contain all or most of the elements in Table 4.1.

**Table 4.1**  Parts of a book

| Part | Explanation |
| --- | --- |
| Foreword | Usually written by someone other than the author. It normally explains how and why the book came to be written and may commend its particular strengths. |
| Preface | Similar to the foreword but written by the author and states the book's origin, scope, purpose, plan and intended audience. In a second or subsequent edition the preface may highlight improvements or changes in content. |
| Introduction | An overview of the content, purpose or scope of the book and how to use the specific book. Usually written by the author. |
| Acknowledgements | A list of people or organizations that the author wishes to thank. This may consist of a dedication. |
| Contents page/s | A contents page will often have sections and chapter titles; a comprehensive contents page will also provide paragraph headings. |
| Index | Probably the most important part of a book as it lists all the important terms and concepts contained in the book in alphabetical order. |

### Foreword/Preface/Introduction

All of these parts of a book do a similar job by providing a quickly read overview of the content. Ten minutes spent reading the introduction will tell you if the book is likely to be useful for your specific purposes.

### Contents page

After the index the contents page is probably the next most useful way of saving time. Contents pages range from basic one-line chapter headings in monographs to sections divided into chapters which are further divided into headed paragraphs. Textbooks are not meant to be read from cover to cover as they are designed to be referred to. Chapters may build on previous chapters, as in this book, but some edited monographs have chapters written by individual authors that could be treated as essays or articles and read individually. Chapters can, of course, be read out of sequence according to your needs as a reader. Contents pages may go into great detail, allowing the reader to locate relevant information quickly.

## Index

While most monographs cover specific subjects or ideas in great depth, a good index is the way to quickly get to the information you need. An index allows the reader to go straight to the pages that they are interested in without flicking through the entire book or chapter. A good index will give the range of pages where the required subject can be found, will redirect the reader to broader or narrower subject terms and give technical alternatives to commonly used terms. Using the index can be equated with using SatNav and is usually a great time saver. Notice the strict alphabetical order in which information is presented in the following example of a book index:

**Kidney** (*Main term*)
 **ageing changes 48, 49** (*Changes to the kidney due to ageing on pages 48 & 49*)
 **disorders SEE Renal disorders** (*look for 'Renal disorders' in the alphabetical list of main terms*)
 **function SEE Renal function** (*look for 'Renal function'*)
 **structure 611–12** (*you will find 'kidney structure' on pages 611–612*)
**Kidney transplantation** (*Main term*) 637–41
 complications 640–1
 nursing care 639–40

N.B. The explanatory notes in brackets do not appear in the index.

## Exercise 4.1

If you have not done so already, take about 15 minutes to examine the book you are reading.

- Compare this book against the parts described in Table 4.1
- Can you detect how early chapters have more relevance for the first year or beginning of your course?
- Test the index by thinking of a topic you would expect to find in a book on study skills – how easy was it to locate the relevant pages using the index?
- Does it appear to be able to meet your needs?

## Effective reading strategies

A common experience when reading is to pause and think:

- 'I don't know what I'm reading!' or
- 'I have hardly taken in any of this so far!'

This is most likely because you have been reading passively without concentration because you do not have a deliberate plan or reading strategy.

When you are familiar with parts of a book this provides a strategy to help you decide if the book is what you want.

- Read the Foreword/Preface/Introduction
- Check chapter headings
- Look for your subject in the index

If it is not what you really need, look for a better, more specific book.

### Skimming or diving deep?

When reading you will have to decide exactly how much information you need from the text. If you only need the most basic of information you can use the strategy described above. If you require more information then you will need to scan the book or text.

### Scanning

- Read the chapter headings and descriptions in depth
- Read any chapter summaries or introductions in depth
- Pick out keywords and concepts mentioned in the text
- Look at illustrations and diagrams; a picture can be worth a thousand words and should never be ignored

### Speed reading

Speed reading is a technique that enables the reader to quickly pick out the relevant blocks of useful information from any irrelevant text. To be an effective speed reader you will need to know what information you want from the text before you start reading. This technique is most useful if you require only basic facts. If you need to understand the content in some depth then you should use another strategy (see SQ3R below).

Speed reading consists of:

- reading the text in blocks, rather than as individual words
- practising improving the number of words you read in each block
- avoiding going back over a previously read block by using a card to follow the text

## Active reading

Active reading is a technique for more in-depth study of a text. It involves high-lighting or underlining relevant passages in the text, but this technique can only be used if you own the text! With e-books and some web pages it may be possible to highlight the text on screen.

What do you do?

- If you do not own the text or do not want to cause damage to your own text, then photocopy the relevant text or cut-n-paste if you are dealing with web pages
- Slowly read the passage and highlight or underline the relevant points
- If you have obtained a copy you can make notes directly onto it

## SQ3R explained

This technique, a more structured form of active reading, allows you to gain maximum benefit from reading a text (Martin, 1985). It can be applied to a book, chapter, journal article, in fact any form of text. As you follow the five sequential steps in this technique, you can develop a mindset into which you can fit the facts. SQ3R stands for Survey, Question and the 3 R's are Read, Recall (or Recite) and Review.

What do you do?

- Survey – quickly scan the chapter headings, watch for diagrams, highlighted text, introductions, summaries and conclusions.
- Question – what information do I need? What information do I already know? Does this text, e.g. chapter of a book, meet my needs? What does this diagram tell me? Jot down a series of questions that arise from your survey, e.g. 'What is the key role of the nurse in caring for a patient following kidney transplant?' 'In view of age related changes in the kidney, how is renal failure defined – is this also age related?
- Read – as you read the text you should be trying to answer the questions that you posed, carefully separating the facts from the waffle. If you answer the questions in your own words it will force you to 'translate' the text into information that you will understand. This makes sure the process is mentally active.
- Recall – you should be able to recite each question you have set and verbally answer it in your own words. Attempt this following the reading stage and make brief notes which answer your guiding questions.
- Review – using the notes you have made rapidly check with the text that your answers are accurate and in the detail you require. To assist in understanding

and memory, plan to mentally go over the information after 24 hours. Review your answers again after a week and repeat until the information sticks in your mind.

## Exercise 4.2

- Find a block of text, a short section from a book, (perhaps the following section headed 'Effective note taking'), an A4 printed paper or short journal article.
- Select a strategy from those outlined above and apply it in reading the material.
- Repeat using a similar *but different* block of text and use a different strategy.
- Compare their effectiveness and consider any differences from your usual method of dealing with text.
- Discuss this with a 'study buddy' and plan to try these strategies in the future.

## Effective note taking

Note taking can be used as part of an effective reading strategy but is most commonly associated with lectures. While lecturers may talk at a rate of 120–240 words per minute, students are capable of taking notes at a rate of only around 20 words per minute. Digital recording of speech and indeed video is increasing so that some of your lectures may be available as podcasts or MP3 files on course-related websites. Yet the need to be able to capture some of the main facts or ideas in your own words makes some form of note taking necessary. However 'it is quite common for people to take vast quantities of notes, to file them away and never look at them again' (Terry, N.D.: 20), so it is important to develop skill in effective note taking if they are to have value after the event.

## Listening

Before you can become an effective note taker you must be an effective listener. There is a real difference between listening to the words and listening to what is being said.

Reasons for not listening effectively include:

- fatigue, a problem often solved by good time management
- losing interest in what is being said
- being so interested that you cannot wait to add your contribution
- spending time thinking of ways to argue against what is being said
- not asking questions if you do not understand
- making judgements about the speaker
- filtering what is being said with your own personal beliefs or biases
- distractions from various sources.

Note taking may be an utter waste of time if it distracts you from listening. At university you are in control of what you learn so in order to produce effective notes you will need to prepare. Find out in advance if possible what you are expected to gain from the lecture. There may be 'outcomes' published, if so obtain these and read them. Prepare by thinking about the title of the lecture in advance, doing some preparatory reading and exploring unfamiliar terminology. Refer back to the section on 'Getting the best from your course' (see Chapter 1). Also consider the value of using SQ3R for lectures which may at least prepare you with some questions that will certainly focus your listening.

Look and listen for:

- lists of points, for example words like 'firstly', 'most importantly', 'note that . . .'
- non-verbal pointers like facial expressions and changes in tone of voice
- time spent on emphasizing a point
- introductions, conclusions and examples from practice.

There are key advantages if you develop the skill of paying special attention to these cues.

## Overview of note taking

- Take the necessary equipment.
- Do not even attempt to record everything that is said.
- Use paper with margins on both sides – this allows for the left part of the page to be obscured by the ring binder folder and space for your marginal notes on the right.
- If you are proficient in shorthand then use it. If not consider developing your own unique shorthand using key abbreviations. You may use R to indicate 'Research' when taking notes in a research module. 'Le' may indicate 'Legal aspects'. To make clear that they are abbreviations you could circle them.
- Note questions. I use the right-hand margin and circle the capital Q. You can then pose these at an opportune time. Alternatively your questions may form the basis of follow-up activities.

Above all, your notes need to be useable if they are to complement your learning and revision. They must not be too cluttered, so leave much blank space on the page.

**Use headings**
By structure
Layout
Space
Show importance of topics.

Highlighter needs to be used consistently but quite sparingly, a page with 80% of the text covered in fluorescent yellow highlighter hardly assists in drawing my attention to the key points!

## Cornell System

This system of note taking was developed at Cornell University to save students rewriting their notes. How is it done?

- Preparation – using paper divided into two columns (see Table 4.2)
- During the lecture
  - write clearly in paragraphs
  - only use abbreviations if you will remember them
  - try to capture facts, ideas and points
- After the lecture go through your notes to
  - fill in blanks
  - check their accuracy
  - make sure they are legible
- Then identify key concepts, thoughts, ideas and facts and write these in the column on the left

**Table 4.2** Cornell note taking system

| Recall column | Note taking column |
| --- | --- |
| This column will contain: | This column will contain the notes taken at the lecture |
| Keywords | Write legibly |
| Summaries | Put down broad concepts, ideas, facts or points |
| Phrases | Use abbreviations |
| Ideas | After the lecture go through the notes and add your own comments, highlight key points and box core ideas |
| Facts | |

# Mind maps

Mind maps are a way of making conceptual links using diagrams instead of using notes. Tony Buzan originally developed the idea, in his book *Use Your Head* (Buzan, 1974). The human brain works in an 'associative' rather than a 'linear' way, so remember what was said at a lecture by making links between words, ideas, illustrations, not by recalling every sentence the lecturer says. Often during lectures and tutorials students will ask for a sentence or phrase to be repeated word for word, passively transferring a set of words from one person to another. Yet it will be more productive to note the ideas in your own words. Mind maps allow you to make notes in the same way as your brain works.

What do you do?

- Using a blank sheet of paper put the main concept in the centre of the page
  - It helps if you print the words and circle them
  - The clearer and stronger this image is, the easier it will be to remember
- Create linked circles for the main ideas, themes, theories, concepts or keywords that link to the central theme
- Use single words or short phrases and emphasize them with underlining, colour or symbols.

Using visual displays such as mind maps as your method of note taking may not always be possible during the lecture. While some lecturers will give a visual or verbal overview as an introduction, often the ways in which knowledge is structured and linked may not become apparent until the lecture is well under way. In this case the production of a mind map will form a useful way of consolidating what you have learned and reduce the amount forgotten if carried out soon after the event. See Figure 4.2.

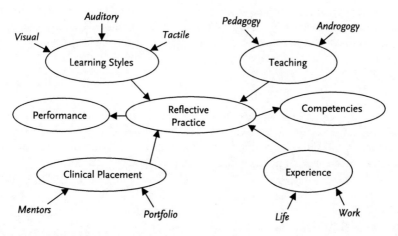

FIGURE 4.2 Mind map

# Writing an essay

Mind maps may also be a very useful strategy in planning an essay. An essay is a piece of writing which is written to a set of conventions (Cottrell, 2003:151). While these conventions may seem odd, and there are sometimes good reasons to deviate from them, it is important that you become familiar with these:

- written in a formal, academic style
- written in the third person – which excludes direct reference to you as the author of the work, 'I', 'me' etc. generally do not appear
- gender is usually written out of the prose
- addressed within stated limits – the set 'task' is bound by a prescribed remit
- objective, concise and precise expression of ideas in the form of an argument
- follows a recognized structure.

However, some of these conventions will be inappropriate in forms of writing such as 'reflection' (see Chapter 5).

## Academic style

Compare the following short sections from an essay on the topic of patient assessment.

> I will ask the client about their own perspective on their current difficulties in coping when I make my assessment and I will also ask his family and any other significant individuals for their views. I think it is important to seek corroboration from others when there are delusional elements in what he says to me.
>
> (56 words)

> The assessment should include the client's own perspective on their current difficulties in coping along with the views of their family and any other significant individuals. It is important to seek corroboration from others when there are delusional elements in what is being presented.
>
> (44 words)

Notice:

- Style; how are the people *(writer, nurse, client, family)* referred to?
- Compare each example using the few details about academic conventions listed above. Which one conforms most closely to these and why?

- Around 20% difference in the word count
- It may be worth reviewing this exercise when you have completed the section on essay writing

### Task analysis in essay writing

Task analysis can be defined as identifying a series of actions, activities and cognitive processes (thoughts), which must be undertaken to accomplish a set task. Any activity such as writing an essay is best understood as a series of tasks. Each task can then be broken down into a series of sub-tasks or actions. By breaking things down into small bite-size pieces it will make the overall task less daunting.

A vital prerequisite for writing an essay is to understand the remit.

### *What is the question?*

Essays are usually written to demonstrate the level of subject knowledge or expertise that you have gained from a module, lecture or course. So the title will usually contain a question, the subject matter to be covered and an indication of the level and type of answer expected. You may be invited to devise your own question, in which case you may need the advice and approval of your lecturer.

When you analyse the title you have to decide what question is being asked, what subjects, concepts, ideas you will need information on and what keywords or subject terms you need to search for. Look out for any of the words in Table 4.3 because they indicate how you should approach the answer and whether it is expected to be descriptive, analytical or critical. These concepts are explained in more detail in Chapter 8.

### *What do I need to answer the question?*

You will need to ask yourself a few questions. What do I already know? What information do I already have? What information do I need to find? Where will I find the information?

### *Are there any gaps?*

Look at the essay title and brainstorm all the words, ideas and thoughts that may relate or link to the question being asked. Use lists to remind you of possible search terms or a mind map to graphically organize your thoughts.

**Table 4.3** Words used in essay titles

| Word | What it means |
|---|---|
| Account for | Give reasons for, clarify, explain, justify |
| Analyse | Examine the concepts, ideas or subject in depth |
| Argue | Make your case for or against a point of view using relevant evidence |
| Compare | Look for similarities within concepts, ideas or subjects (see contrast) |
| Contrast | Look for differences within concepts, ideas or subjects (see compare) |
| Define | Make a precise statement about an issue, idea or concept |
| Describe | Give a detailed account of an issue, idea or concept |
| Discuss | Give reasons for and against an issue by argument |
| Evaluate | Using the work of others weigh up the arguments surrounding issues |
| Illustrate | Use examples to clarify an issue, idea or concept |
| Outline | Present the main issues, ideas or concepts within a subject area |
| Review | Make a list of everything available on a particular subject |
| Summarize | Give a brief description of the main issues, ideas or concepts |

## Getting the information

You will already have some information in notes taken from any lectures you have attended. You may have also been given a reading list to support the module. You will also have to incorporate some unique information gathered from a literature search (see Chapter 6). When you have gathered your information you will have to sort it into highly relevant, quite relevant and irrelevant. Once completed, you can then start taking notes from the most relevant material.

Once you understand the overall task you can now begin to engage with each sub-task in turn.

## Exercise 4.3

It is so important to have an accurate analysis of the task when it comes to essay requirements that if it were possible to compel readers and students to undertake one exercise from this chapter, this would be the one.

- Form a syndicate of students who have an identical essay task set
- Agree to work independently and then join together to discuss your task analyses

- Highlight key concepts within the given title and write out your understanding of these terms in one or two sentences
- List ideas and topics which you feel MUST be covered in the essay
- When these stages are complete meet with your syndicate group and share your conclusions
- Where there are differences discuss these fully
- Remember that essay titles give a general indication of the requirements, each person's essay can and must be quite different
- Anything which remains unclear must be the topic of a discussion/email question to the person who set the question, your academic supervisor or equivalent lecturer.

Once this is clear you have firm direction to proceed with the subsequent stages or sub-tasks in the preparation of your essay. The essay must be structured and ideas expressed should logically follow in developing your thesis. Table 4.4 outlines recognized parts of an essay but you must adhere to the prescribed format set by your lecturers.

## Thesis and argument

An essay could be described as an objective, concise and precise expression of ideas in the form of an argument and 'an academic argument is a claim or proposition put forward, with reasons or evidence supporting it' (Masterson, 2005:192). This is by no means implying that you should be *argumentative* in your assignments, but that methodical reasoning to support your points must be presented logically, often in a calm and objective way. The term 'thesis', sometimes referring to a particular academic assignment, implies essentially the same ideas as an academic argument, being a proposition to be maintained or proved.

The idea of evidence is central; types and strength of evidence and critical thinking are examined in more detail in other sections of this book, but it is worth considering the elements of academic argumentation here.

### *Components of an argument*

- Your point or position is clearly stated
  - Maintaining very close observations on a designated patient in acute psychiatric nursing ('special' observation) is counterproductive
- An explanation of the reason for your point is given
  - This infringes humans rights, agitates people, exacerbates paranoia and ultimately does not prevent self-harm
- Evidence to support your claim is presented
  - Research has shown that immediately after this level of observation is relaxed patients have committed suicide (add reference to relevant research)

**Table 4.4** Parts of an essay

| Essay part | What it should contain |
| --- | --- |
| Opening statement | This is usually one sentence outlining your argument or thesis and the broad direction it will take |
| Introduction | Can be one or several paragraphs introducing your argument or thesis in detail |
| | It should be used to lead the reader into reading the rest of the essay and should usually be around 10% or less of the permitted wordage |
| Body | This is where you bring together facts, citing or quoting appropriate sources, examples and other information to make your argument or forward your thesis |
| | It forms the bulk of the textual information in the essay. You will need to address several issues or make several key points |
| | **Point 1** (state and amplify) |
| | Back up with evidence, explaining relevance to the question |
| | Connect with |
| | **Point 2** (state and amplify) |
| | Back up with evidence/indicate opposing argument |
| | Proceed with as many points as required |
| | Links between points must be made explicit |
| | Often in midwifery and nursing you will also need to make explicit links to some aspect of professional practice |
| Conclusion | This briefly summarizes the essay and reiterates the main points of arguments you have made |
| | The conclusion contains no new material |
| | Ensure your conclusion really is that – that you have mentioned the points in your essay |
| | Make sure the conclusion relates to the essay title |
| Reference list | This is a list of all information sources or references you have quoted or paraphrased in your essay |
| | Your university will have a policy regarding references that you should refer to |
| | Readers should be able to find the sources you have used |
| Bibliography | Some universities require a list of all the information sources you have read yet not cited in addition to the reference list |
| | Words contained within the bibliography, along with those in the reference list, are generally not counted in any word limit |

It is important therefore that you decide on your position, the points you wish to make and then make a strong argument well supported by evidence presented in plain English. Redman (2006) in his very useful book on essay writing suggests that you consider your reader to be someone at the same level as yourself in another university. Assuming this level of knowledge frees you from explaining every detail and gives more space to develop your arguments.

Where work is presented which consists of strings of quotes or where students fear expressing their own position, it may be judged to be of poor quality precisely because of the lack of argument. It is worth considering the way in which you incorporate references in your text here.

## Exercise 4.4

Read the following extracts from an essay.

Community homes for people with learning disabilities are a failed attempt at social integration because of NIMBY syndrome, fear of the unknown and endemic discrimination.

(Bloggs 1988, Smith 1997, Patel 2004).

Patel (2004), who has undertaken many community studies on behalf of the Disability Rights Commission, suggests that extensive preparation for community-based group homes is essential if any degree of social integration is to be achieved.

Reflect on which is more common and which is most impressive and why?

The examples are entirely fictitious but they serve to illustrate some important points. While the 'Bloggs, Smith and Patel' approach may impress some, and indeed this is the way many students and some academics write, it may simply amount to 'kite-marking'. Canter and Fairbairn (2006), both experienced academics and authors, strongly oppose the 'kite-marking' approach to citations. It may look impressive, it may indicate you have done some reading but the reader is not informed about the quality of the source, nor in the example above, which point is being supported (or opposed) by which author. We strongly advocate what we call the 'value-added' approach as illustrated in the second example above; you are informed about Patel and his or her work and affiliation.

Discuss this with your peers and your lecturers in relation to work you are undertaking.

## Self-checking of your essay draft

At the stage where you have an early but fairly complete draft of an essay or other academic piece of written work it will be useful to review your progress against the following check list:

- Seriously consider the comments of a 'critical friend' if you have someone taking this role.
- Read the draft with the following questions in mind:
  - How is this relevant to the title?
  - If I were not the author of this essay would the relevance of my points be extremely clear?
- Are your main points made explicitly? i.e. what is your position on the issues?
- Are you using evidence to logically support the points you are arguing?
- Using highlighter pens and your own colour coding, go through a clean draft and mark sections against important criteria which reflect the academic level and requirements, e.g.
  - describes   (pink)
  - applies knowledge to the topic   (green)
  - analyses the issues   (yellow)
  - justifies the points I am making (evaluation)   (blue)
  - This will then show at a glance the balance of features and, depending on the exact requirements, whether there is a need to alter the balance in the draft you are working on. N.B. A draft that is mainly pink is likely to need considerable improvement.
- After making changes, re-read your introduction to ensure it still reflects both the remit and what the essay has developed into. Alter this if necessary.
- Check that you are conforming to the required referencing system and tick each reference on the list as you read it in your draft – detail must match precisely.

# Conclusion

This chapter has argued that studying is most efficient when it is active and deliberate in applying strategies that can improve your effectiveness for successful learning. People with recognized learning disabilities are encouraged to develop additional strategies and make use of reasonable adjustments that universities make. Strategies for reading, note taking and essay writing have been outlined but these will be of little value unless you make a conscious effort to try them and persist in developing skill and confidence in their use. If you have skipped the exercises, especially the one promoting accurate task analysis related to essay titles, you have not yet finished this chapter. While this may not be problematic to you, so much rests on this you are strongly urged to ensure your strategies are not undermined by poor task analysis. Your course is likely to be demanding but with good time management and the use of strategies outlined here, you will find that these demands are not beyond your grasp.

# 5

# Reflective learning in clinical practice

*Introduction • Patients: our teachers • Mentors and other support in practice*
*• Relationships • Assessor role • Care pathways and learning pathways*
*• Learning pathways • Reflection: learning incidents and models • Critical*
*incident analysis • Reflective models • Professional portfolio • Coping with*
*practice • Conclusion*

This chapter considers the particular needs of qualified nurses and midwives undertaking CPD courses, but initially concentrates on introducing undergraduate nursing and midwifery students to the array of learning opportunities provided by clinical practice settings. First among these will be patients or clients receiving a service in their placement areas, arguably the single most important source for learning. The supervisor or mentor is a very significant person amongst others: colleagues from other disciplines, social workers, dieticians, police liaison officers, doctors, operating department practitioners, physiotherapists and drama therapists; each have a role in assisting your learning. Many placement settings have a well-established and clearly structured set of both 'care' and 'learning' pathways which will be examined with a focus on their potential for learning. 'Reflection' on learning incidents is explored along with reflective models and the professional portfolio. Finally pointers for coping and surviving placements are given.

# Introduction

Learning from clinical practice is the most exciting part of the course yet for some it is the most daunting. Contact with patients is the reason for applying for the course in the first place; many do not initially appreciate the value of university-based learning and cannot wait for the first placement allocations to go onto the notice board, or more likely the course website. For the qualified nurse or midwife this all seems easy, they deal with clinical demands every day displaying admirable skill but to the novice learner observing their proficiency it may seem well beyond their grasp. Yet just a few years ago many of these same nurses or midwives were taking their own first tentative and fearful steps into the clinic, the labour suite, the patient's own home or the hospital ward, going through similar joys, anxieties and agonies that the new student feels.

Qualified staff may not view their clinical practice as a place for learning, at least not to the same extent as pre-registration students, though most respond to their professional obligation to engage in learning throughout their entire careers. Some continuing professional development (CPD) courses undertaken after qualification have placements away from students' normal place of employment. However, most courses direct these nurses and midwives to their own clinical practice as rich sources of learning. Practice settings are increasingly valued as places for learning from the range of experience students are exposed to. However, it is the pre-registration undergraduate nursing and midwifery students who will need most preparation for this part of their courses if they are to get the best from their practice placements. Clinical practice placements are where you will be allocated to join the established staff, share their rotas and duties and meet patients, clients, service users, and well people as well as very sick people. Yet in some situations the term 'clinical' will initially appear to be quite inappropriate, e.g.

- group home for five people with learning disabilities
- drop-in centre for people with long-term mental health difficulties
- undertaking checks on the newborn infant and mother in her own home
- nursery run by a charity in an inner city area.

These hardly meet the criteria for the label 'clinical' yet undergraduate midwifery and nursing students, from various branches, will find that they have fairly lengthy placement in just such areas. And each provides valuable learning opportunities, supported by supervisors within areas where nursing and midwifery are legitimately practised. In fact there is a considerable move to locate many health services outside acute hospital settings. Even when people are quite acutely ill they may still be cared for in their own homes via 'hospital at home' or 'home treatment service' schemes for acutely sick children or people with acute mental illness. Reflection is a concept familiar to nurses and midwives and soon to take on particular significance to the undergraduate student in these fields as it relates very much to learning from experience. It will soon become apparent that reflection is a massive subject within nursing and midwifery, which is integral to clinical practice and lifelong learning. Its treatment here will be more than sufficient to get you started and feeling comfortable with reflective learning and writing.

# Patients: our teachers

I listened recently to a talk by a respected ornithologist and theologian, who with great insight, enthusiasm and many clear illustrations, explained how much humans have to learn from birds. This was both fascinating and enlightening yet imagining the idea that people can learn from birds could be viewed as incredible. A similar reaction may occur in relation to the idea that patients may be our teachers. Nurses and midwives have cared for and taught countless patients and this is much easier to accept: that the qualified practitioner has a role in teaching their patients. However, with little experience most students could come up with quite a list of things that the nurse or midwife teaches:

- antenatal classes
- strategies for coping with depression
- walking with the aid of elbow crutches
- how to manage pain in childbirth
- taking medication for childhood asthma using a spacer device
- instillation of eye drops.

Those qualified, however, could fill a book (London, 1999) with things that make up their responsibilities to teach; yet the clients dealt with and the patients cared for may also act as our teachers.

Whether our meeting with them is on day one of our first clinical placement or after 30 years experience, patients are often our teachers. Most patients would not conceive the idea that they have anything to teach us, quite the reverse in fact. Nevertheless in our normal dealings with clients there is much to learn about them as individuals and they can provide essential lessons. Patients inadvertently provide triggers for our learning and these will be diverse, leading nursing and midwifery students to many areas of knowledge such as psychology or skills such as administration of medications. Some triggers will challenge our long-held beliefs and attitudes, such as the role that smoking may play in helping women cope with the pressures of child rearing responsibilities (Graham and Blackburn, 1998).

## Live lessons

While students must *learn about* communication, more importantly they may *learn to* communicate in different situations. And it is patients who may teach these skills. Learning about the path people have taken to arrive at their current situation as 'patients', how they got to the stage in their lives where they are seeking or receiving a service from health professionals, including nurses or midwives. And since this relationship first occurred, giving and receiving a nursing or midwifery service, what has the experience been for the one on the receiving end?

Learning about the psychological impact on a 14-year-old boy or 36-year-old woman of having to adjust to surgery creating a colostomy, now residing on the surface of their abdomen, and changing and emptying the bag of faecal material (McKenzie *et al.*, 2006). Adjustment and changes in body image are subjects found in textbooks and undoubtedly these are of great value in learning about related psychology. However, such patients will teach us live lessons and our learning becomes complete and relevant. Patients are our teachers because they have been through illness, treatment and other experiences while the nurse or midwife has not.

## Expert patients

Beyond the inadvertent 'patient as teacher' whereby nurses, midwives and students learn from patients by recognizing encounters for their educational value and make efforts to make the most of these, some patients are seen as 'expert patients' and take on the role of teacher more formally. People live with their own treatment regimens for many decades; they are attuned to their own bodies and minds and can accurately detect and interpret quite minor changes and adjust their own treatment or consult the nurse or doctor in time to prevent deterioration or complications. Some become more knowledgeable than the average nurse or midwife so that it may be foolish to dismiss what the diabetic lady tells the midwife about the state of her diabetes at a key stage in her pregnancy.

In recognition of the fact that so many in the population live with some form of chronic illness, e.g. more than 8 million people in the UK are affected by a neurological condition (Neurological Alliance, 2004) and around 27,000 people under the age of 27 have arthritis (Arthritis Care, 2006), the National Health Service set up the 'Expert Patients Programmes' in 2002. These consist of short courses for patients who are taught how to live and cope with their illnesses and how to more effectively engage with health and social services. The Expert Patients Programmes do not concentrate on any specific long-term condition, they do encourage and teach the skills patients require to become self-sufficient in seeking specific information. These people are soon able to focus on their own needs, understand what they can reasonably expect and therefore become more discerning consumers. They take on 'self-management'. Patients may then take a more formal role in teaching health professionals, and a more assertive stance in their normal interaction with health professionals.

While this may appear quite radical and challenging, particularly to the novice learner who may enter nursing or midwifery with the traditional view that the professional knows best, there are many positive spin-offs. Such patients are likely to make appropriate use of the health services, be focused on what they want and be fairly clear about what they need. This would naturally lead to better efficiency with less staff time diverted on unnecessary actions. The relationship nurses and midwives are able to develop with such patients will continue to be on the basis of the provision of a service but the learning opportunities for nurses or midwives are enhanced.

Some fields of nursing have a history of valuing patients for what they have to teach experienced staff and new students. Students on a learning disability nursing course will have clients involved in classroom activities and even interviewing candidates for the course. In clinical practice this ethos continues and is set to become much more widespread as policies are eventually translated into practice (Department of Health, 2004a; Gillam and Brooks, 2001). Public and patient involvement in all aspects of health care, including nursing and midwifery, designing services, evaluating services and associated education programmes, is a key strategic goal which supports the notion of the patient as teacher.

The term 'patient journey' is familiar to some nurses such as those working in oncology where the notion 'cancer journey' has particular significance. It is something patients can teach us in most fields of practice. It may not be possible, and may be dangerous, to generalize from just one patient's experience. However, discovering 'patient journeys' will enable you to appreciate the sort of milestones, setbacks, lows and highs that people go through as they negotiate the health and other systems over the course of their particular journey. There will certainly be some applications from engaging with such patients when later faced with similar circumstances and faced with searching or difficult questions from our future patients and their relatives.

## Patients' rights, learners' obligations

There are of course issues that need consideration relating to confidentiality, ethics, tact and genuine respect for people in a patient role when they are often quite vulnerable. The Nursing and Midwifery Council have produced some guidance specifically for students (Nursing and Midwifery Council, 2002) that makes clear that patient information remains personal, private and confidential. Where it is necessary to refer to patients in written assignments, they make it clear that you must not 'provide any information that could identify a particular patient' (Nursing and Midwifery Council, 2002:5). Clearly learners must become familiar with university policies and may need to take advice from mentors or other senior colleagues and above all make sure that patients are not exploited or insensitively viewed as objects for learning. While most patients are content to have contact with students and may themselves benefit from this (Ely and Lear, 2003) the NMC make it absolutely clear that 'Their rights as patients supersede at all times your rights to knowledge and experience' (Nursing and Midwifery Council, 2002:4). Yet not to exploit the opportunities presented by our experiences with patients for our learning is wasteful of an essential ingredient in the process of becoming a qualified nurse or midwife. If the services offered are to become increasingly responsive to patients' needs, be it in the acute psychiatric setting or as a school nurse, any CPD student cannot afford to neglect the patient as teacher. Many learners report that it was their contact with patients which was the key to their real understanding; where there is application of theory or research findings to professional practice, learning becomes so much more meaningful. Some incidents will be so novel and momentous that they give rise to 'flashbulb memories' (Eysenck and Keane, 2005:274) and where you see the relevance of live lessons long-term memory is enhanced, patients are valued and future practice is enhanced.

In viewing patients as teachers students must:

- respect patient's wishes in any potential learning situation and seek their consent, especially where you wish to observe a procedure
- let patients know the capacity in which you have contact with them
- be tactful and ensure you are aware of the patient's current situation; discuss this with a supervisor or mentor
- talk to patients and more importantly listen to their stories
- acknowledge your own limitations in terms of skills or knowledge
- respect what they say and use this to trigger further learning.

## Exercise 5.1

First identify what 'patients' are referred to in your placement.

What title is designated as appropriate will soon become apparent by listening to practice-based colleagues.

Now reflect and then discuss with peers and experienced nurses, midwives or other members of the multidisciplinary team using the following trigger questions:

- To what extent is this form of address expected by clients?
- Does this promote an 'us and them' situation adding to professional distancing?
- Are there benefits to staff or patients inherent in this?
- Does this reveal much about the real philosophy of care in operation in your placement area?
- How does the title designated as appropriate in your field differ from others?
- How may clients cope with the transition, e.g. when transferred from adolescent to adult services or an ITU to a surgical ward?

To mirror the variation of forms of address this book uses a range of terms.

# Mentors and other support in practice

As you begin to undertake placements the importance of the mentor and other key individuals who offer support to learners in practice will soon become apparent to you. Colleagues and friends will begin to enthuse about how great their mentor is, how excellent their placement is and how much learning is being achieved. CPD students will also be involved with clinically-based colleagues, most of whom are experienced practitioners with a key role to facilitate and assess practice-based learning.

It will be helpful to all students therefore to be clear, in advance, about the role and responsibilities of the mentor, what can reasonably be expected, policy and standards published by the Nursing and Midwifery Council, and how to make the most of the professional relationship your course places you in.

A mentor has been defined as 'an advisor'. This may be a friend advising over a protracted time span on career development. People who have achieved notable rank within their field of work, be it a chief executive or the president of the Royal College of Nursing, will often cite key individuals who have supported them or guided and encouraged them: a mentor. In clinical practice the role has come to be seen as a qualified practitioner who takes some responsibility for supervising learners over a relatively short period. The learner is likely to have little or no say in their selection.

The Nursing and Midwifery Council (NMC) have recently updated their standards in relation to this key role to support learning in clinical practice (Nursing and Midwifery Council, 2006a). An NMC mentor is someone on the NMC register who, following successful completion of an NMC approved mentor preparation programme, has achieved the knowledge, skills and competence required to meet the defined outcomes.

Such mentors are deemed responsible and accountable for:

- organizing and coordinating student learning activities in practice
- supervising students in learning situations and providing them with constructive feedback on their achievements
- setting and monitoring achievement of realistic learning objectives
- assessing total performance including skills, attitudes and behaviours
- providing evidence as required by programme providers of student achievement or lack of achievement
- liaising with others (e.g. practice facilitators, practice teachers, personal tutors, course directors) to provide feedback and identify any concerns about the student's performance and agree action plans as appropriate
- providing evidence for, or acting as, sign-off mentors with regard to making decisions about achievement of proficiency at the end of a placement or part of the programme (Nursing and Midwifery Council, 2006b).

The university will keep a live register of mentors who meet all the specified criteria and they are responsible along with placement staff for providing you with a mentor. Local arrangements are usually in place to ensure that shift patterns, holiday and sickness will not leave you without a mentor but you may liaise with more than one designated mentor on a placement.


# Relationships

At a recent conference designed to update mentors, the head of a nursing home for people with long-term mental health problems described her current student on placement. The first year mental health student made it very clear that she does not like old people, she hates reading and she can't abide learning. Neither the best start nor the most positive impression to project to one's mentor! One key relationship during practice-based learning is the one between the student and the mentor. In addition to the CPD qualifications the designated mentor has achieved, their formal relationship with a student entails a considerable amount of work, and often this is in addition to their own clinical caseload. A mentor is a significant person and a good relationship must be something you strive for.

This will be enhanced if you take the initiative and

- ring and visit the placement in advance to meet your mentor
- plan and avoid any possible hindrance to arriving on time for every allocated shift
- display a professional business-like approach; you are there to learn
- consider any reasonable request and acknowledge that you may learn by doing

- demonstrate appreciation of the work and goodwill involved in taking the role of mentor
- present neat and clear documentation for discussion and signing off.

## Assessor role

In spite of some concerns over possible role incompatibility, this same person will play a major role, hopefully with others, in making judgements about students' progress. They will decide whether the student has reached the required standards, demonstrated competence or achieved the specified practice outcomes, or not. While many others from outside midwifery or nursing contribute towards your learning from practice, and may be able to verify your achievements, it is only the designated mentor who can sign off whole outcomes within practice grids or other practice-based assessment documentation provided by your university.

## Care pathways and learning pathways

While you will be taught that patients are individuals they share some common experiences with others. Indeed some will follow similar pathways throughout an episode of care involving many different health professionals. 'Care pathways' have been introduced across the NHS for many patient situations. In recognition of the inter-professional nature of most patients' needs these have come to be called integrated care pathways (ICP). The following defines ICPs and illustrates their aim for quality standardization: 'Integrated care pathways are structured multidisciplinary care plans which detail essential steps in the care of patients with a specific clinical problem and describe the expected progress of the patient' (Campbell *et al.*, 1998).

ICPs, which carry their own documentation, have been devised for a wide range of patient conditions and situations such as:

- oral health care of people with learning disabilities
- deliberate self-harm
- fractured neck of femur
- elective caesarean section (see National Health Service, National Library for Health, 2005 for further details).

As a student or CPD learner you will become familiar with ICPs which should ensure that everyone who participates in the pathway does so knowing what happens at earlier and later stages of the care a particular patient receives.

While ICPs are important in their own right they also provide a ready-made structure to guide many aspects of reflective learning within clinical placements. Pollard and Hibbert (2004) describe 'placement pathways' inviting students to follow patients within an ICP, an experience often augmented by the requirement for students to achieve objectives and give an account of these to their mentor. Crucially this includes the need to identify positive impact for future patient care. One such account followed a student's visit to theatres to observe open abdominal surgery. Her appreciation of postoperative pain reported by patients changed dramatically as a result. Feedback from this project shows that senior staff and students found it useful and it is 'a good way to use supernumerary status' (Pollard and Hibbert, 2004:43).

# Learning pathways

Some universities, working closely with associated practice-based partners, have devised comprehensive 'learning pathways' for many placements.

The 'learning pathway' is an innovative concept of learning that aims to provide students with insights into the patient's journey through the health care system as well as facilitate an appreciation of the various roles of the multidisciplinary team members that the patient may be exposed to during their journey. It also provides links mapping the pathways of learning to:

• clinical learning outcomes required by the specific course
• learning needs related to the stage in the course, e.g. year one or year three
• National Service Frameworks related to the placement
• 'Essence of Care' benchmarking guidelines from the Department of Health (Department of Health, 2003).

The model used may be 'hub and spokes', whereby the placement location itself becomes the hub, providing around 80% of the learning opportunities with other pathways, represented by the spokes, which takes students to various departments, key staff or clinics. So the majority of time is spent within the confines of the placement area, while the remainder may be with specialist colleagues accompanying clients on their ICP. Hub and spokes may therefore be distinguished conceptually as:

home-based placement    peripheral staff of departments
basic care    advanced care
uni-professional    inter-professional (non-nurses/non-midwives).

An illustrative example of a hub and spokes model is provided in Table 5.1.

Specific documentation for students may accompany each practice placement outlining the learning pathways and options available which include space for notes, reflective comments and specific questions designed to enhance the application of learning that has occurred such as:

- What have I learnt?
- How can I apply this in my clinical practice?
- How can I share what I have learnt with my colleagues and/or the clients and families that I care for?
- In what ways can this learning influence my forthcoming role as staff nurse or midwife?

Many placements have a very clear menu of learning opportunities. It is worth noting that you bring your own life experiences, knowledge and personal characteristics which can significantly contribute to patient care. Your presence in placement will stimulate mentors and other clinically-based colleagues to learn themselves.

**Table 5.1** Learning pathway on a urology ward placement

| Hub: designated 'basic' | Spokes: more advanced learning opportunities |
| --- | --- |
| Patient hygiene | Urodynamics |
| Privacy and dignity | Flow rate |
| Confidentiality | Prostate assessment |
| Self-care deficit | Penile erectile dysfunction |
| Pressure relieving care | Catheter change clinic |
| Nutrition needs | Extracorporeal shockwave lithotripsy (ESWL) |
| Tissue viability | Bladder instillation |
| Infection control | Haematuria clinic |
| Care of a deceased patient | Flexible cystoscopy |
| Support of relatives | Follow-up clinic |
| Continence, bladder and bowel care | |
| Clinical observations | |
| Record keeping | |
| Handling and moving | |
| Oral care | |
| Wound management | |

# Reflection: learning incidents and models

The concept of 'reflection' has been commonplace in nursing and midwifery for around two decades, and rather than turning out to be a passing fad among educationalists, it has spread to all fields of education and practice and well beyond health-related courses. Nurses and midwives have embraced reflection, reflective practice, reflective learning, models of reflection and reflective writing.

As with most concepts there is some scope for ambiguity. When re-learning to brush one's hair after a stroke a mirror provides essential reflection. For mental health nurses reflection is essential to effective communication when talking to a client with severely altered mood or in a counselling situation, whereby they may reflect the posture or feelings of the client.

Reflection, in terms of learning from experience (and this is not necessarily confined to clinical practice settings) is a concept that has been the subject of a glut of academic and professional papers, conference presentations and books. And while it may be viewed primarily as a tool for learning and professional development, nurses and midwives may have to write assignments which focus on the concept or tool itself as well as having to utilize the tool for learning! Critical examination of the subject will reveal that it may be viewed as a complex, contested, under-researched and perplexing phenomenon that is hard to explain (Burns and Bulman, 2000:3).

Qual' ʳurses and midwives, perhaps depending on the number of years si⁻ may not immediately see the need to become reflective practi- ⁻s can recall when things were very different and some ᴧerished, their passing bemoaned passionately. Clearly all ᴠ to be beneficial with hindsight, and there is at times more things have always been done. Traditional practice was char- ᴧct hierarchy within the grades or ranks of nurses with just the charge nurse assuming responsibility. The day was divided up by ᴧtients might have multiple nurses attending to distinct aspects of . And as many a nurse or midwife will tell you, all the work was com- ᴧo a high standard! Practice was something to be completed with efficiency ᴧn activity from which to learn. This emphasis, utterly familiar to those who ᴠerienced it was from an era characterized by:

- The importance of routine; theatres were cleaned by nurses at weekends
- Ritualism, the consultants ward round commanded near silence from staff and patients
- Discouragement of questions: like Victorian children, the student's place was to remain quiet and do as instructed

- Discouragement of displays of emotion: if a very sick child died the nurse was to remain composed at all times
- Skills explained by intuition, gut feelings or personal experience-based practice prevailed without question.

Since around the late 1970s or early 1980s this situation has gradually changed and continues to evolve as nurses come to accept their legal and professional status of individual accountability. Coupled with this is an increased awareness of the value of the Social Learning Theory (Bandura, 1977) in explaining how learning is promoted by observing social situations such as working with mentors. The approach which characterizes reflective practice is one of

- improvisation, dealing with novel situations
- a spirit of enquiry, inquisitiveness and questioning as acceptable and encouraged
- research based, being able to justify ones practice with reference to robust evidence
- experiential teaching, deliberate and planned within formal curricula
- feelings shared and explored, acknowledgment that these impact on practice
- our abilities to cope and an acceptance that on occasions, support may be necessary
- knowledge-based skills, being able to rationally explain skills.

In practice reflection is sufficiently understood and finds much appeal within nursing and midwifery and can be defined as 'deliberately thinking or mulling over experiences with the intention of learning'. Although writers on this topic examine reflection-in-action (Burns and Bulman, 2000:3), implying that the process occurs in real time, during professional practice spanning just a minute amount of time, the main focus here is what has been conceived of as reflection-on-action. Reflection-in-action may relate to experienced staff, with well-established knowledge and skill in a particular field of professional practice. However, even the experienced midwife or nurse in a learning capacity during CPD studies, will be focused on learning from novel situations. Lincoln et al. (1997:100) distinguish reflection from mere experience and assert that 'there can be no true growth in learning by mere experience alone, but only by reflecting on experience'.

A strategy of 'deliberately thinking or mulling over experiences with the intention of learning' or reflection-on-action in this context is viewed as an activity which is:

- retrospective
- contemplative
- structured

- probing
- a trigger for learning
- cognitive
- purposeful
- emotional
- cyclical.

Primarily reflection is retrospective, occurring as a private cognitive activity in the mind of the person, for our purposes a student or learner. Perhaps the process is best started soon after the event or experience to minimize recall bias or loss of detail. Maybe as a result of checking with others the thinking process is extended and reflection becomes more public: student to mentor 'That patient who refused his medication from me, yet took it after you spoke to him, what exactly did you say about the side effects?'

With the answer comes a more accurate and comprehensive understanding of exactly what happened. Equipped with this the student may then contemplate utilizing their current knowledge but may come to realize that additional knowledge would help her learning from this experience. Reflection is therefore a trigger for probing beyond this starting point and, in this example, may lead to further activities. The student may look up the drug/s in question or consider professional self-image and persuasive communication. She may re-read the local policy and consider ethics and rights of the patient to accept or refuse his medication. Furthermore she will recall the record keeping requirements and after recovering from the initial feeling of rejection when the patient refused her attempts she may decide how to approach similar situations in future.

Here the student has drawn on many topics during the process of reflection, which may have occurred over several days involving an Internet search, chat with colleagues or mentors and some reading. In effect this potentially incorporated a direct or indirect application of knowledge from:

- pharmacology and reporting side effects (yellow card system)
- anatomy, physiology and pathology
- law and ethics
- rights and responsibilities
- communication and interpersonal skills
- role modelling, imitating the actions of competent colleagues
- record keeping.

Learning could then be identified and the learner completes the cycle when faced with a similar situation: the approach she had decided upon is tried out in practice and the results of this are then subject to deliberately thinking or mulling over this new experience with the intention of learning. It may be that the approach was effective, but if not the cycle of reflection starts again.

# Critical incident analysis

As novice learners soon discover, nursing and midwifery is awash with abbreviations and terms that are alien to the average outsider. Qualified colleagues are not of course outsiders and these present fewer difficulties but in entering a new arena, the world of professional education, this advantage may be lost. The term 'reflection' provides one such example and the related concept 'critical incident analysis' provides another. However, the experience outlined in the previous section provides an easily understood explanation because it was an incident from which the student learned. They learned because they deliberately thought about and carefully weighed up this experience with the explicit intention of learning; they used reflection as a tool for learning.

'Critical incident analysis' has several component parts. Analysis is to examine carefully and break down component parts of a situation; the incident is the experience itself and the term 'critical' is used since it was critical for the student's learning. It may be clearer to omit the term critical since it is the cause of some confusion. A learning incident is then simply the event, experience or incident that is subject to analysis and the analysis may take the form of reflection. Learning incident analysis becomes the central event which the reflective process is applied to.

Learners with limited experience may come across practice during their placements where it appears that the standard of practice is poor. After reflection however a quite different interpretation may emerge. A note of caution must be sounded here; one that will be supported by your university documentation. While lessons must be learned from poor standards of professional practice that come to light, students should avoid selecting such incidents for their formal educational requirements. You are accountable and required to act on what you observe where it may amount to unprofessional conduct. Your mentor, the host organization, your university and the Nursing and Midwifery Council offer advice to staff and students in these circumstances but an assignment is not the place to report concerns.

# Reflective models

Not surprisingly, reflection, as a logical and clearly structured process of thinking, has been described by numerous writers who have proposed models to outline and simplify the process for those who wish to understand or use it. A model may help us to appreciate how the parts of the process fit together and is supposed to represent reality. There are of course models of nursing, models of disability, which fit the category of a 'conceptual model'. To assist the process of learning from clinical practice, or any type of learning incident, there are models of reflection. While you may at some point need to examine or compare and even write about reflective models, the purpose of this section is to outline just two possible models and their utility value. You will certainly need to use reflection and there is no doubt that using a model will make the process more efficient. Many students must also demonstrate the use of a model of reflection to pass the course of study. This topic will therefore be revisited in Chapter 9 where reflective writing is considered in relation to assessments.

In essence reflection may lead to improved patient care through application of the learning which occurs, as pointed out by Basford and Slevin (1999:113), 'The process of reflection occurs within a cyclical framework requiring the practitioner to reappraise the care given and in so doing analyse and evaluate the effectiveness of that care'.

Reflective models show the cyclical nature of the process and many have similar stages and starting points, often concluding with action planned as a direct result of learning. They are nothing more than loose guides to assist and structure the process, and will be especially helpful when you are unfamiliar with reflective learning or where you wish to commit the thought processes to paper.

A reflective model introduced by Johns in 1994 is fairly typical (see Figure 5.1). This writer sees the stages simply as cues to help learning from experience and these are sequentially as follows:

- description
- reflection
- influencing factors
- alternative strategies
- learning.

This model could help the student who had been involved in the example cited earlier where a patient initially refused medication. It provides a structured way to deliberately think or mull over this experience with the intention of learning from it.

Atkins and Murphy (1994), however, proposed a model which starts with 'discomfort' and would therefore be more appropriate in circumstances where the experience or incident was initially characterized by some form of discomfort (see Figure 5.2). As a student in the learning disability branch you may visit a family in their own home and hear how the child with a form of autistic spectrum disorder returned from her mainstream school distressed by the alleged behaviour of her peers. It is revealed that the class teacher has been unsupportive and other parents have made derogatory comments to the child's mother at the school gates. Suppose your initial reaction was a feeling of discomfort, this incident may best be explored with the aid of Atkins and Murphy's (1994) model of reflection using each stage as follows:

- feeling of discomfort
- description of events + thoughts and feelings
- analyse feelings and knowledge
- evaluate its relevance
- identify learning
- action/s.

### Exercise 5.2

- Select an incident which has triggered your learning recently
- Review Johns (1994) cues for learning and the stages suggested by Atkins and Murphy (1994) and decide which of these models to utilize

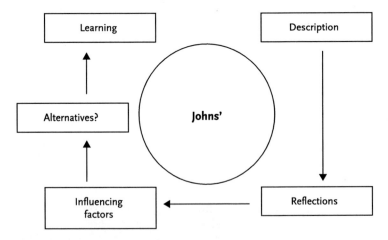

**FIGURE 5.1**  Reflective model by Johns (1994)

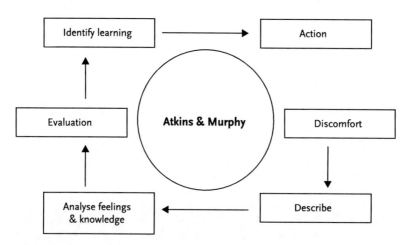

**FIGURE 5.2** Reflective model by Atkins and Murphy (1994)

- Make brief notes to match each of the headings within the model related to the learning incident
- Discuss this process with your mentor, peers or personal tutor
- Bear in mind the alternative strategy or actions you have decided on for use in similar clinical situations
- Consider making a written record of this exercise, perhaps in your professional portfolio

# Professional portfolio

Formally introduced by the English National Board for Nursing, Midwifery and Health Visiting, a now defunct part of the governing body superseded by the Nursing and Midwifery Council, the use of a professional portfolio is a well-established requirement. It is a private document compiled by individual nurses or midwives, bringing together records of achievement. Most students will be required to use a portfolio and if not it is strongly advised to start keeping such a collection for a variety of reasons.

One of the first writers on this topic within nursing and midwifery described a portfolio as 'a private collection of evidence which demonstrates the continuing acquisition of skills, knowledge and attitudes, understanding and achievement. It is both retrospective and prospective, as well as reflecting the current stage of development and activity of the individual' (Brown, 1995:2). Amongst many other things it may contain your reflective accounts showing your individual learning from incidents. As such many of the entries may be confidential and personal. In view of this a related term has been used to describe those sections which the owner of the portfolio selects and chooses to make public, perhaps for a particular purpose. Then the selection may be referred to as a 'profile', which is a selection of specific evidence for a specific purpose for a specific audience (Hull and Redfern, 1996).

This purpose may be for an interview or in compiling a CV for an application for a new post or course or it may well be educational in nature. You may extract sections of your portfolio, i.e. a profile to bring to a seminar you are presenting to colleagues, to a tutorial or in some courses a profile may be the designated method used in assessment. While there are commercially produced documents designed for this purpose, your university, the NHS or another employer may provide you with a document or template, most likely in electronic format. Pebble Pad is one such format and while it may be initially supplied as part of a course, students may continue to utilize this web-based portfolio well beyond the completion of a formal course. In this case the student has the ability to make sections open to any Internet user should they so wish.

# Coping with practice

Most qualified nurses and midwives have developed their coping skills and survived many traumas. Undertaking a CPD course however may well bring additional traumas and added stressors, bringing you closer to the fine line between 'stimulating and exciting' and stress or not coping. For the novice student or student in year three the demands of learning from clinical practice are almost inevitably going to feel overwhelming at times. Demands from patients and relatives, peers, mentors and university assessments can at times bring their unique emotional and psychological pressures on top of other obligations adult students feel. The result will occasionally be a sort of mental paralysis characterized by reduced ability to think clearly or prioritize.

It may just help to know that most people have been there at some point and the normality of this situation may empower you to acknowledge the issues and seek help. A key to coping here is to acknowledge that you feel there is a problem.

It is possible to reflect on the incident if your feelings originate from an incident and indeed learn from that, but in the middle of what could amount to a crisis of confidence, it may just be the wrong time to employ this strategy.

The traumatic experiences you will undoubtedly be exposed to are just that; traumatic. A 32-year-old mother, diagnosed as brain dead, is being visited by her two small children to say their farewells in an intensive care unit prior to enacting the clinical decision to switch off the ventilator. Also there is the demand to deal with competing extremes almost simultaneously. A joyful patient and his family have just received news that a donor, a 32-year-old woman, has been found and preparations for his life-saving liver transplant must begin immediately. Perhaps your supervisor or mentor will demonstrate admirable coping skills in such a situation. If so seek their advice. Those with direct or indirect involvement, including yourself, will have a variety of perspectives on these traumatic events. Examining these in informal discussions holds the potential for learning for all involved.

Expressing emotions such as crying may be seen by some as a departure from the designated nurse or midwife role, but relatives after a death in coronary care reporting that the nurse cried took this as a comfort and a sign that he cared so much.

The particular circumstances may have impacted on the wider team of practice-based colleagues, for example where there is a suicide amongst the client group. In this case there will be both formal and informal mechanisms whereby staff are supported and you should tap into these resources.

## Pointers for survival

- This is common and normal
- Crying is also normal, this may be the time and the place
- Peers, friends and family are likely to be very supportive
- The current situation is very likely to be short-lived
- Others have coped with similar stressors and many are willing to support you
- Courses do have built in safeguards to ensure temporary difficulties do not hinder achievement of the required outcomes
- A few days away from the practice placement area may be legitimate
- Chaplaincy or counselling services are available either through the placement organization or the university
- Personal tutors or course directors will be able to help or direct you to key sources of help
- You must develop your own coping skills and the situation you are in will be instrumental in this development
- Hold onto the belief that this is going to be helpful to you in future

## Conclusion

Developing skill and confidence in reflective learning from practice is just as essential as other study strategies for all nursing and midwifery students. These are prerequisite for developing competence for practice and making the most of the lifelong learning opportunities daily contact with patients affords. Whilst patients and mentors may be excellent teachers and the placement offers a rich menu of learning opportunities it is your attitude and engagement with reflective practice which is key to sustainable learning. Familiarization with the use of reflective models will certainly help to structure this important part of the course where theory and practice merge in live learning situations. The three years will bring a catalogue of incidents, some very traumatic. Even these can serve you well in enabling you to develop emotional resilience, a quality at least as important as cognitive abilities or practical skills to ensure successful study and practice as a midwife or nurse.

# Part 3

Becoming competent: advanced learning for nursing and midwifery students

# 6

# Literature searching skills for midwives and nurses

*Introduction • Aims of a literature search • Getting started • Search strategy • What am I searching for? • Terminology in a search strategy • Keywords versus subject headings • Subject headings • Subject tree • Keyword searching • Using terminology • Database field searching • Boolean operators • Truncation • Wildcards • Adjacency searching • Nested searches • Limiting a search • Search history • Evaluation • Citations • Study types • Keeping records • Personal bibliographic software • Conclusion*

Literature searching is defined; its aims and associated strategies are explored. Searching by 'keyword' and 'subject heading' are discussed, highlighting the particular characteristics of these tools in effective literature searching. Many other devices or search tools are explained and illustrated which will convince readers of the value of developing these essential skills. Literature is a vast term making it important that nurses and midwives can not only locate literature but be able to evaluate its quality. How to evaluate and record the results of a literature search is covered along with a section on bibliographic software. Most searchers will be used to undertake a 'literature review', a concept which is however covered in Chapter 7.

# Introduction

As a student of nursing or midwifery you may be familiar with the process of gathering information for an assignment using the library facilities and the Internet. If you are not very confident it may pay you to read or revisit Chapter 3, which introduced you to information sources and basic library skills. This chapter will take you one step further and introduce you to the scientific concept of literature searching. Literature searching is an essential part of research methodology in all branches of knowledge. Any proposed research activity should involve a literature search to ensure that similar work has not already been conducted, to see if anyone else is working in the same field or to refine a research proposal using any studies that have validity within the same area of study.

> It is an essential step for researchers to justify any newly proposed research since unnecessary duplication is viewed as unethical.
>
> (Department of Health, 2005)

This extreme position more or less excluded students from learning by doing research. This has been challenged by experienced teachers and students in health care (Corr *et al.*, 2006) but it strengthens the need for good literature searching skills.

Usually when literature is considered, a prize winning novel springs to mind, but what students are looking for is scientific or scholarly literature which comes in varying formats such as journal articles, books, government and technical reports, conference proceedings and web-based scientific publications. Scientific literature is normally peer reviewed by a panel of subject experts or referees to ensure the quality of the information before it gets published in a journal. In essence these publications report or comment on the results of research conducted within the disciplines of nursing and midwifery.

Literature searching can be defined as 'a systematic and thorough search of all types of published (scientific) literature in order to identify as many items as possible that are relevant to a particular topic' (Gash, 1989:1).

In order that important information is not overlooked a literature search must be undertaken using a systematic methodology. So knowing what you are not looking for is as important as knowing what you are.

# Aims of a literature search

- To determine what has been published in your field
- To identify potential relationships between research concepts and practice
- To determine how others have defined key concepts and applied them in research and practice
- To identify key authors, sources and studies that other practitioners refer to
- To ascertain how a body of research develops and how it relates to the work of nurses and midwives in practice

Most students of nursing and midwifery will not go on to become active researchers but they will need to be cognisant of the value of, and role that, research plays in underpinning developments in practice and patient care. Most nursing and midwifery students will undertake a literature search, from a different perspective from that of the researcher although their reasons will sit within the general aims of a search.

The reasons nursing and midwifery students undertake a literature search include professional development or current awareness purposes and to:

- find information for an assignment/dissertation/thesis
- support evidence-based practice
- find out if others are doing similar work to yourself
- provide justification for services or ways of treating patients
- support clinical governance
- investigate a subject of particular interest to you
- aid patient empowerment and awareness.

Clearly the skills involved in conducting a literature search are essential skills for researchers. Midwives, nurses and students from within these professions also need to develop these skills for their own specific purposes.

# Getting started

A literature search may seem a daunting task to undertake particularly if you are new to the idea. If you spend time thinking and planning before making a start on your search it will make the whole process much easier.

## Search strategy

A distinction must be made between a search strategy and a search history. A search strategy is an outline of what you are looking for, what you are going to search, how you plan to undertake the search and what results you are expecting to find. It is your plan of action prepared in advance. A search history is a list of terms and actions undertaken during a search of an individual database that can be saved and re-used.

A systematic approach to planning, recording what has been searched, and what needs to be searched, ensures that all relevant resources are used. Figure 6.1 outlines the procedures that are undertaken during the course of a search.

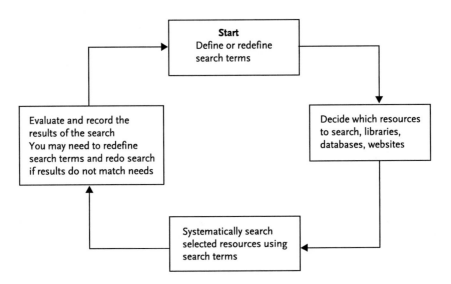

**FIGURE 6.1**  Search strategy

## What am I searching for?

The topic of a literature search will often be an assignment that forms part of the assessment of a module undertaken at university, so the subject will be closely defined. Some topics for searches will be decided jointly with a lecturer while others you will have to decide from a list of alternative subjects. If a topic has been closely defined the extent and level of the search has to be decided upon. A novice student would be expected to find references from a reading list and some supporting information. While a final year student would be expected to independently find and synthesize information to support an argument developed within an assignment.

Before considering the topic of a search it is important to think about the types of information you may require. For instance if you are considering the implications of a change of government policy on an aspect of clinical practice you would need:

- government reports
- policy documents
- comments or opinions of practitioners.

This would require a search of the library catalogue, government websites and databases and most of the results would be found in reports or policy documents. Whereas if you were considering how an aspect of clinical practice has been improved by the application of research findings you would need to search databases, systematic reviews and look at relevant clinical guidelines and most results would be found in journal articles.

If you have not been set a topic for a search one of the most difficult tasks of literature searching is deciding what you are looking for. One way of making the process easier is to formulate a search topic using the PICO methodology. The PICO methodology was originally designed to formulate research questions but it can be employed to enable you to identify the elements needed to define your search terms (Stone, 2002).

- Patient population, condition or disease
- Interventions (diagnostic or treatment)
- Comparisons
- Outcomes

For example you might decide that the subject of your search will be an examination of the problems associated with the prevalence of pressure sores on an elderly care ward. See Table 6.1.

Being more specific you could decide for example that you are going to find information to compare the performance of various types of bed or the difference between turning the patient and the type of bed used for the reduction of pressure sores. So your topic could be written as follows: 'A comparison of the

**Table 6.1** PICO method

| P | I | C | O |
|---|---|---|---|
| Pressure sores | Wound care, beds, turning | (beds vs beds), (types of bed vs turning), (wound care vs types of bed), (wound care vs turning) | Treatment, prevention or reduction of pressure sore incidence |

performance of various types of bed and patient turning to reduce the incidence of pressure sores on an elderly care ward.'

## Exercise 6.1

The mother of an adolescent child with a learning disability is becoming increasingly concerned about her child becoming obese and asks you for advice. How would you frame the search topic from the information you have received from the child's mother? Use the PICO chart in Figure 6.2 to help you.

Think carefully about the factors that may address the obesity problem.

| P | I | C | O |
|---|---|---|---|
|   |   |   |   |

FIGURE 6.2  PICO chart

# Terminology in a search strategy

When you are conducting a search the way you use language is as important as it is in everyday communication. For instance if the word 'awful' is used today it means terrible but when used in the 17th century it would mean amazing because the original meaning was 'full of awe' or 'awful'. There are a number of things that need to be taken into consideration when deciding on the terminology to use in a search. It is a good practice to record the terminology used in a search and add to it as the search progresses and more terms are identified. Once you master some of the peculiarities of literature searching terminology it will make the process more efficient.

# Keywords versus subject headings

Many students assume that keywords and subject headings are interchangeable concepts. They are in fact very different and both have a specific function to play in a comprehensive literature search.

Take the words 'pressure sores'; if a keyword search is conducted on a health database it will retrieve a number of relevant references. However, the search will have missed a lot more relevant references because the following terms were not also searched:

- pressure sore
- pressure ulcer
- pressure ulcers
- decubitus ulcer
- decubitus ulcers
- bed sore
- bed sores.

If searching by keyword all of the options above would have to be searched separately in order for the search to be comprehensive because it will only retrieve data containing the exact terms you have used, that is 'pressure sores'. Keyword searches tend to be an inefficient method of searching a database and their exclusive use may lead to a false assumption that you have retrieved a comprehensive list of references.

# Subject headings

Most health databases also have the option to search using subject headings. Subject headings are a controlled language (or thesaurus) designed to reflect the subject content of the reference irrespective of the words used. Subject headings are decided by subject experts and allocated only if they are relevant. So a search using the subject heading 'pressure ulcer' would find references using any of the above terms without you searching for all the alternatives separately. Notice the immediate saving of your time!

MeSH (Medical Subject Headings) from the National Library of Medicine is the most commonly used system in medicine whilst CINAHL subject headings have been designed to reflect the needs of nurses, midwives and other health professionals. Key concepts are used in both sets of headings for consistency. Using a set of standardized headings to categorize the subject content of references is also useful in the construction of a subject tree. A subject tree allows the searcher to either broaden the search to wider terminology or narrow the search to more specific terms. If you look at the diagram of a subject tree below, skin diseases would be the branch while pressure ulcer would be the twig!

# Subject tree

Skin and connective tissue diseases (widest term – all related diseases)
    Skin diseases (just skin diseases)
        Skin ulcer (all types of skin ulcer)
          Pressure ulcer (specific term)

Most health databases have a facility to map (or compare) the word or words you type to a list of preferred headings. So if you typed 'bed sores' it would give you the option of using the preferred MeSH heading of 'pressure ulcer' or stay with the keyword search of 'bed sores'. Some databases will do this automatically each time you search whilst others have a separate search facility for subject headings.

From the topic 'A comparison of the performance of various types of bed with patient turning to reduce the incidence of pressure sores on an elderly care ward' you will need to identify those terms you think will be subject headings. It is a good idea to ignore words like comparison, performance, types, reduce and incidence which have a broad meaning and could be applied to anything. Concentrate on words like pressure sores, beds, patient turning and elderly that have a specific meaning and are more likely to be subject headings or search terms.

# Keyword searching

A search using a subject heading will retrieve most references but it may not retrieve them all and there are some online resources that do not have the facility of searching subject headings. When you are searching a database it is worth considering using keywords in addition to subject headings if the search has to be comprehensive.

When constructing a list of terms for a search every variation of the term both wider and more specific should be used. Jargon and natural language phrases should be avoided or used as a last resort unless it is the only information you have. You can search for popular or jargon names such as Viagra and look at the subject headings to find the chemical name of sildenafil. A search using the subject heading of sildenafil will find you far more relevant references. Using natural language to search for 'National Service Framework' you will retrieve references that contain the phrase. It is always beneficial to check the retrieved references for the allocated subject headings. You can then undertake a further search using those subject headings to retrieve more useful references.

## Exercise 6.2

Using your search topic from the previous exercise you will now need to identify relevant search terms. Make a list of all of the alternative terminologies used for learning disabilities. Then do the same for the other words in your search topic.

# Using terminology

When keyword searching the word variations in Table 6.2 should be taken into consideration.

**Table 6.2** Search terminology

| Term | Meaning |
| --- | --- |
| Synonyms | different words with similar or identical meanings |
| Antonyms | words with opposite or nearly opposite meanings |
| Homonyms | words spelled the same but with different meanings |
| Alternative spellings | pediatric or paediatric, oedema or edema |
| Plurals (p) | diagnosis(s) diagnoses(p), bacteria(s) bacterium(p) |
| Natural language | searches using everyday phrases |
| Jargon | the special language of a certain group or profession |

# Database field searching

A database is made up of references that are further divided into fields. A field is a category of information that the database can search such as the author's name or a journal title. Many of the fields can be searched independently. The examples shown in Tables 6.3 and 6.4 are normally used but it is worth checking what is used on the database you are using. This can be done using the Help function that can be found on all databases.

Field searching can be a useful strategy especially if you are keyword or natural language searching. A search conducted using 'National Service Framework.ti' will find only references with that phrase in the title of the reference, while a search using 'National Service Framework.ab' will find all references with this

**Table 6.3** Example of a database record

| Fields | Database bibliographic record |
|---|---|
| Author | Tzeng Y |
| Title | Enema prior to labor: a controversial routine in Taiwan |
| Source | Journal of Nursing Research. 2005 Dec; 13(4): 263–9. |
| Subject headings | Enema, episiotomy, labor, induced |
| Abstract | The results of this study indicate that the administration of enemas as a routine practice prior to labor is not substantiated by medical necessity. |

**Table 6.4** Database search fields

| Field Name | Searches | Examples |
|---|---|---|
| .ab or .AB | for a word in the abstract | labor.ab |
| .au or .AU | for an author | tzeng,y.au |
| .jn or .SO | for a journal title | journal of nursing research.jn |
| .su or .MH | for a subject heading | enema.su |
| .ti or .TI | for a word in the article title | labor.ti |
| .tw or .TX | for a word in all searchable fields | administration.tw |
| .pg or .PP | for a page number | 263.pg or 263.PP |

phrase in the abstract. References containing the phrase in the abstract are more likely to be evaluative than those with the phrase in the title which are more likely to be comments or opinions.

# Boolean operators

George Boole (1815–1864) invented the concept of Boolean algebra, which formed the basis of computing and information technology. Boolean operators allow searches to be conducted using more than one concept. Concepts can also be combined within, or excluded from, a search. The three Boolean operators AND, OR, NOT, allow searches to be broadened to find more or narrowed to find fewer references.

For example a search using the search terms identified earlier in the example topic (pressure sores AND beds) would find references containing both search terms. A search using (pressure sores AND (beds OR patient turning)) would find references with either (pressure sores AND beds) or (pressure sores AND patient turning), while a search using (pressure sores AND (elderly NOT adults)) would find only references about pressure sores and elderly (see Table 6.5).

Table 6.5 Boolean search operators

| Boolean operator | Search examples | Searches for |
| --- | --- | --- |
| AND | triage AND child | both search terms in a reference |
| OR | child OR infant | either search term in a reference |
| NOT | child NOT infant | references excluding the search term 'infant' |

# Truncation

Most databases allow words to be truncated or shortened using a symbol to replace the missing letters. This allows a searcher to find references containing words with the same beginning or stem. You may wish to find references containing any of the following search terms: midwife, midwifery or midwives. In such a scenario a search could be conducted employing the phrase (midwife OR midwifery OR midwives) using the Boolean operator OR. However if midwi* was used the same references would be found using the short cut of truncation. There is also a facility that allows you to limit the number of letters after the stem so a search for nurs$2 would retrieve only references containing the words nurses or nursed. This allows a search to be widened, resulting in more references being retrieved.

# Wildcards

Wildcards are similar to truncation in that symbols are used to substitute letters within a word. The symbols allow searches for both the singular and plural forms such as woman or women using either wom#n or wom?n. Wildcards are also useful when searching for variations in spelling. For example when searching for paediatrics you would also need to include the American spelling pediatrics. Using wildcards you could simultaneously search for both using the form p?ediatrics.

# Adjacency searching

A keyword using heart attack will search the database for heart, attack and heart attack with the result that more irrelevant records are retrieved. Such a search would include references to the anatomy of the heart in human and non-human species. It would also retrieve all references containing the word attack in whatever context the word was being used. However the same search using heart ADJ attack or 'heart attack' will find the exact and complete phrase. An adjacency will also search for phrases by using a positional indicator. For instance a search for 'client ADJ5 relationship' will find 'nurse client relationship', 'client nurse relationship' or the 'relationship of the nurse to the client'; as long as client is within five words of relationship any phrase containing those words will be found.

# Nested searches

Many search engines and databases allow nested searches to be undertaken. Nested searches are complex searches using both Boolean operators and brackets.

Operations are prioritized with those in the brackets being performed first followed by those functions outside.

Using the example topic a search could look like this:

- (pressure sore* AND (bed* OR mattress*))

If the above example of a nested searched was typed into a database all the operations listed below would be undertaken simultaneously thus saving time. See Table 6.6.

**Table 6.6** Nested searching

| Operation | Search for | Results |
|---|---|---|
| 1 | Bed or beds | 200 |
| 2 | Mattress or mattresses | 100 |
| 3 | Either bed(s) OR mattress(es) | 300 |
| 4 | Pressure sore or pressure sores | 6000 |
| 5 | All references containing:<br>pressure sore(s) AND bed<br>pressure sore(s) AND beds<br>pressure sore(s) AND mattress<br>pressure sore(s) AND mattresses | 75 |

# Limiting a search

One common experience many students face when undertaking a literature search is that an enormous amount of references are retrieved. There are two ways of reducing the number of references retrieved from a database search. The first is to combine more than one concept in a search, but care should be taken if more than three concepts are used as the search may retrieve very few references. The second way of reducing the number of references is by applying limitations to the format of the reference. For instance you may wish to retrieve only reports of case studies relating to patient restraint published in British nursing journals in 2004. See Table 6.7 for common limitations used in databases.

**Table 6.7** Search limits

| Types of limitation | Limits references retrieved to? |
| --- | --- |
| Publication year | A particular year or range of years i.e. 2006 or 2007–2008 |
| Language | English, French, German, Japanese |
| Age group | Fetus, infant, child, adolescent, adult, aged |
| Latest update | References added to the database within the month |
| Journals subset | Nursing, health promotion/education, peer reviewed etc. |
| Review articles | Classic review articles |
| Research articles | Classic research articles |
| Publication type | Case study, clinical trial, practice guideline, etc. |

# Search history

A search history is a record of the terms and actions you have used when searching a database. Most databases allow you to set up your own space where you can save a useful search history and reuse it. So for instance you could save the search history below and run it on the database every month. This would retrieve any new clinical trials published within the month and is known as a current awareness search.

Table 6.8 demonstrates an exhaustive search for nursing-based clinical trials of beds, mattresses or cushions used to prevent pressure sores.

## Exercise 6.3

Having constructed a search topic and identified a list of search terms and their alternatives, you are now ready to undertake a search on a database. Select a relevant database from those you have access to. See if you can construct a search history using your search terms. Use the one in Table 6.8 to illustrate the techniques you may wish to employ in your search.

# Evaluation

When you have conducted a literature search you will need to evaluate the information you have retrieved in case it does not answer the question you have set. If it does not answer your question you may have to re-evaluate your search

**Table 6.8** Example of a search history

| Set | Search term | What does it mean? |
| --- | --- | --- |
| 1 | Pressure ulcer/ | Subject heading search |
| 2 | (pressure ADJ (sore* OR ulcer*)).ti,ab | Nested keyword search of titles and abstracts |
| 3 | Decubitus ADJ ulcer*.ti,ab | Keyword adjacency search of titles and abstracts |
| 4 | 1 OR 2 OR 3 | Boolean search combining all the alternatives in sets 1, 2 and 3 |
| 5 | Beds/ | Subject heading search |
| 6 | Mattresses/ | Subject heading search |
| 7 | Bed*.tw | Truncated keyword search |
| 8 | Mattress*.tw | Truncated keyword search |
| 9 | Cushion*.tw | Truncated keyword search |
| 10 | 5 OR 6 OR 7 OR 8 OR 9 | Boolean search combining all the alternatives in sets 5, 6, 7, 8, 9 |
| 11 | 4 AND 10 | Boolean search combining all variations of pressure sores and beds/mattresses/cushions |
| 12 | Limit 11 to clinical trial and nursing journals | Looks only for clinical trials in nursing journals |
| 13 | Limit to latest update | Finds references added to the database in the last month |

terms and adjust your search strategy to include a wider range of resources. For example if you were conducting a search for the 'ethics of using restraint procedures in learning disability nursing' on a nursing database and you did not retrieve many references, you could broaden the search to include medical, psychological and social studies databases, but you should also reconsider the search terms you used in the search.

If you did retrieve references to meet the needs of your topic you would still need to evaluate the quality of the information. While the skills needed for critically evaluating the content of individual research articles will be covered in Chapter 7, it is worthwhile to develop the ability to sort retrieved references by their relevance and level. The indicators in Table 6.9 can help you decide whether the reference is worth considering.

**Table 6.9** Evaluating search results

| Look for | |
| --- | --- |
| Abstract | If a reference has an abstract it is more likely to contain substantive information<br>References without abstracts tend to be comments, letters or opinions |
| Pages | The number of pages a reference contains indicates whether it is a substantive article<br>Single page references also tend to be comments, letters or opinions |
| References | The higher the number of references referred to in an article gives an indication of the quality and coverage |
| Citations | Many databases include an indication of the number of times an article has been cited or used in other reference lists<br>If an article has been regularly cited in other articles it is regarded as high quality |
| Journal | The title of a journal containing the article also gives an indication of the quality of the information<br>You are much more likely to find research-based information in an academic journal than a popular title |

# Citations

A citation search is an advanced search technique that enables searchers to identify key authors, sources and studies that other practitioners refer to. If you already have a substantive article, a citation search will allow you to find references published later that have cited the original article. However, articles are cited for a number of reasons in addition to actually using the information in the original article to write further articles. So care should be taken when using citation searches for the following reasons:

- Articles are cited as part of the critical appraisal process for criticism or comment
- Authors can cite their own work to increase their prestige
- Authors often cite articles by members of the journal referees panel
- Citations may be left out because of word limits on submitted articles
- Colleagues often cite each other's work
- In some disciplines journal literature is not the main medium of communication

# Study types

Within the disciplines of medicine and health, different types of research study are designed to answer discrete research questions. When undertaking a literature search consideration of the design of the research study can be used to assess the validity of the content of retrieved references. See Table 6.10.

**Table 6.10** Research study types

| Research type | Example | Study type |
|---|---|---|
| Effectiveness of a policy, procedure, intervention or therapy | Would a nurse-produced patient education leaflet reduce asthma readmission rates in children with asthma? | Clinical trial Controlled clinical trial Randomized controlled trial |
| The likely pattern or outcome of a condition, disease or health problem | Are post-menopausal women taking hormone replacement therapy more prone to the development of breast cancer? | Cohort study Case controlled study Case study |
| Subjective information such as feelings or perceptions | How do parents of children with Prader–Willi syndrome feel about restrictive diets? | Qualitative studies |
| Which type of diagnostic test or assessment works best | Would health visitors asking primigravida mothers if they felt depressed accurately identify cases of postpartum depression? | Cross-sectional studies |

# Keeping records

You will save a lot of time if you take a systematic approach to keeping a record of what you have done, how you did it and what you found. As part of your search strategy you should record all the search terms used and the resources accessed. You will also end up with a lot of bibliographic references that you have used to make the arguments in your assignment. Most commercial databases will allow you to set up a password protected personal account where you can save your search history and amend or re-use it. Some personal accounts will also allow bibliographic references to be stored.

Most databases will allow your bibliographic references and search history to be downloaded and saved to text files. These can be quickly converted to Word© files and added to your reference lists or bibliographies. If you are working away from your normal computer, your search results and history can be emailed to your computer and then cut and pasted into your Word© files. Reviewing previous search histories can help you define terms for later searches and you may need to re-use a search history to refine and develop your arguments within an assignment.

Students and practitioners undertaking extensive literature searches for research, to meet the requirements of higher level study or if they are writing for publication, may need to use software to store and manipulate the information generated by their searches.

# Personal bibliographic software

Commercial bibliographic software is a product that enables researchers to manipulate and store bibliographic references retrieved during a literature search. These personal databases help with the following tasks:

- They can search for and build a database of references downloading biblio- graphic information from most electronic resources including databases and library catalogues
- They allow citation data to be imported, duplicate references to be removed, data fields to be edited and output sorted numerically or alphabetically to construct bibliographies or reference lists
- They can reformat the information into any preferred citation style required for publication
- Some have additional tools that work with word processing programs to enable citations to be included automatically as you type.

If you are involved in research or are undertaking a literature search for a higher degree it may be worthwhile looking at what software is available to you. The most commonly used packages are Endnote©, Procite© and Reference Manager©. One of these packages may be available in your university so it is worth checking.

# Conclusion

If you invest time and thought to developing your search strategy then you will have a plan to work to. Make sure you identify and use the correct terms to undertake your search. Be aware of which resources to use. If then you do not find relevant references go back to your strategy and look at both the terms and the resources you are using. It is worth remembering that your librarian will always be available to help with both search strategies and selection of resources to use.

Most nursing and midwifery students use a literature search to obtain sufficient information to meet the requirements of the current assignment they are undertaking. They are unaware that they are developing skills that they will continue to use throughout their career. A few student nurses and midwives will go on to become serious researchers undertaking literature searches regularly but most will only use the skills occasionally. When qualified, most practitioners do not notice when they want information on a condition, a procedure, a clinical guideline or a job interview that they are using the skills of literature searching to obtain that information.

# 7

# Proficient use of evidence and research to support nursing and midwifery

*Introduction • Evidence • Context of evidence-based practice • The nature and strength of evidence • Hierarchies of evidence • Research • Classifications of research • Research designs • Reviewing literature • Critiquing research • Issues pertaining to quantitative research • Issues pertaining to qualitative research • Conclusions*

The notion of 'evidence' is examined in the context of 'evidence-based practice' (EBP) as it relates to nursing and midwifery. Clearly all evidence is not of equal value, a view endorsed by the existence of hierarchies of evidence. However, the concept of 'research' and related concepts are presented first to help you gain an appreciation of the nature and strength of evidence.

Classifications and designs of research are comprehensively introduced. Searching the literature, covered in Chapter 6, is developed further in relation to a frequent requirement of courses and professional practice: the need to conduct a literature review. Another set of skills you will have to develop relates to critiquing published research and guidance is provided for critiquing both qualitative and quantitative research.

# Introduction

Recent initiatives have brought nursing and midwifery to its current climate, which embraces the notion of 'evidence-based practice', and requires a reasonably good appreciation of research. Learning about research and the processes involved has evolved within nursing and midwifery to the point where very few, except at higher degree level, will engage in 'learning by doing'. This reflects the ethical concerns of educators and Department of Health policy that most students will have to learn about research by studying research methods, proposing a project, critically evaluating other people's research or writing a critical review of research literature. Where your course supports a learning by doing approach it is important to remain focused on its main purpose which is to learn about the research process rather than the production of some ground breaking new findings. However there will be many positive spin-offs from this approach. The classical dissertation which consists of undertaking a small research project is increasingly being replaced by a 10,000 word literature review or its equivalent.

Whichever way your own course deals with EBP and research, it is vital that you gain sufficient research awareness to become a discerning research consumer, able to understand and use research appropriately in clinical practice. In spite of the concerns the topic of research generates even the most research-phobic student or qualified nurse or midwife can become skilled at appraising the quality of research for their practice. Triggers for reflection on aspects of EBP and professional research are provided and it will be shown that the ongoing proficient use of evidence and research requires many of the skills and qualities of a lifelong learner outlined elsewhere in this book. Your professional commitment to delivering care based on current 'best practice' using appropriate evidence makes these topics essential.

# Evidence

In a court of law a conviction will not be considered 'safe' unless the evidence or the 'facts' presented to the magistrate, judge or jury is both strong and convincing. Hearsay, uncorroborated or weak evidence where there is considerable uncertainty, will not be sufficient to prove or disprove an allegation. There are some high profile cases where new evidence has apparently been discovered changing the outcome entirely.

In nursing and midwifery and health care in general there is a well-established requirement to base our approach to therapies, treatments or 'care' on the best available evidence. The analogy with legal practice is useful since the notion of 'strength of evidence' and the need for 'corroboration' illustrates the situation within health care where the 'evidence' is primarily viewed as research and corroboration equates with the concept 'triangulation' (Canning and Scullion, 2001). Triangulation describes an attempt to confirm research findings by various means. Nurses and midwives must be convinced, and able to convince others, that what they do is safe because of the underlying evidence, and students must learn about the nature and quality of the evidence if they are to make proficient use of it.

The imperative to proficiently use evidence and research is relatively recent. Some nurses and midwives will remember routine practices that have, in the light of new evidence, been shown to be ineffective or even harmful. In the past professional time was devoted to activities and approaches that resulted in no tangible benefits to patients.

## Exercise 7.1

Recall one such practice – students on pre-registration programmes may have to consult experienced nurses or midwives for an example – and consider:

- Who advocated the practice?
- How much did it cost in terms of time, resources, consumables etc.?
- Did the senior members of your professional discipline question it?
- What factors contributed towards its demise?; why is the practice no longer routinely carried out?

The novice student may be alarmed by the revelation that so-called helping professions have engaged in activities that have no supporting evidence. Worse still, that the 'allegation' or assumption that such practices represented safe high-quality care have only quite recently been challenged.

# Context of evidence-based practice

None can escape noticing that the current context in which nursing and midwifery are played out is an evidence-based, research-conscious one. Irrespective of our branch of nursing or midwifery it is no longer acceptable to base our practice on personal preferences alone. 'Without the underlying scientific evidence for them, and a rigorous examination as to their efficacy' (Mason and Whitehead, 2003:325), particular practices may be unethical, unprofessional and unsustainable. Evidence-based clinical practice is an approach to decision making in which the experienced / expert clinician uses the best evidence available, in consultation with the patient, to decide upon the option that suits that patient best.

In each of the following examples the nurse or midwife needs to use the available evidence proficiently:

- attempts to prevent repeat offending by a client with dual diagnosis (e.g. alcohol dependency and mental health issue)
- dressings for different types of wounds (e.g. burn, leg ulcer, dog bite)
- fetal monitoring in uncomplicated labour
- preoperative assessment and preparations for elective orthopaedic surgery, e.g. hip replacement (often carried out in nurse-led clinics)
- psychological nursing interventions to assist the sick child who is reluctant to comply with treatments
- secure fixation of the nasogastric tube for the neonate in a special care baby unit (SCBU)
- the use of reality orientation in the older client who is disorientated and slightly confused.

In these examples and in much of what is carried out, there is an obligation to the Nursing and Midwifery Council to justify our practice and the support for this must be in the form of evidence. To quote directly from the NMC Code of Conduct (clause 6.5): 'You have a responsibility to deliver care based on current evidence, best practice and, where applicable, validated research when it is available' (Nursing and Midwifery Council, 2004a). This sits comfortably in support of policy and professional practice within health care which demands the carefully considered use of current best available evidence, by expert nurses and midwives to patient care situations taking note of the wishes of patients themselves.

## The nature and strength of evidence

There are numerous sources of knowledge or information, which demand our attention and which may direct our thinking and ultimately our professional practice. However nurses and midwives and particularly students with limited experience must be very cautious about which sources they are influenced by.

In decision making there are innumerable 'bits' of information or evidence, which may influence our final decision.

## Exercise 7.2

Pick one of the following situations:

- You want to buy a computer
- Year two is fast approaching and you need different accommodation
- An election is imminent and you have a vote
- A holiday in the sun is planned and you wish to protect your skin.

1 Rapidly write a lengthy list of bits of information that you might consider in making your decision
2 Review your list and cross out those items which you will not be influenced by
3 Number the remaining items to indicate the importance you attach to them
4 Consider the two ends of your scale, most and least important bits of information and reflect on why you have assigned these priorities
5 If you have a 'study buddy' compare the decision making process you have engaged in with them.

This exercise illustrates that there are many sources and types of information. Some information is trusted and accepted while some of it is rejected for various reasons. On occasions when two sources of information are contradictory and without additional knowledge a firm decision may not be made. Clearly personal preference is influential in decision making, as are the views and experiences of friends but the source, nature and strength of evidence are also important considerations.

In professional practice students are sometimes faced with similar dilemmas with competing sources of evidence pulling decision making in opposite directions. Take the situation involving a patient with mild dysphagia (swallowing difficulty) who requests some ice cream. A student will need to be cautious and decline while they seek advice. The qualified nurse or midwife is required to provide a justifiable answer and she may consider all of the following before coming to a decision:

- advice from colleagues such as the rehabilitation consultant or the speech and language therapist
- documented care plan
- professional or legal implications of your action or inaction
- research on dysphagia
- the role of the nurse in conducting swallowing assessments

- the patient's rights and wishes
- your experience and individual knowledge of this patient (i.e. history of choking, presence of diabetes).

In the above example a wrong decision resulted in a nurse being struck off the NMC register in one case (Scullion, 2003).

# Hierarchies of evidence

To assist in the proficient use of information and research, hierarchies of evidence have been proposed. These generally reflect the dominance of a 'scientific' view of reality, which suggests that this is the only legitimate way of knowing. However, nurses and midwives increasingly accept numerous ways of knowing as legitimate which calls into question the value of hierarchies of evidence built on assumptions which are not universally accepted. Qualitative types of research provide invaluable insights about patients or clients which should not be dismissed simply because of the absence of statistical analyses. The theory of knowledge, known as epistemology (Audi, 1998), examines the standards of evidence required to justify believing that things are true. You may need to examine this topic further as your course progresses, certainly in a degree or higher degree course.

In spite of the inherent rejection of some forms of research these hierarchies are very useful when used appropriately to determine the strength of quantitative research studies. See Table 7.1.

# Research

The UK research strategy encourages high quality research specifically to meet the needs of the NHS (Department of Health, 2006a). It supports a public- and patient-centred agenda, a stance which inevitably promotes and explains the focus of funded research projects by reflecting national priorities. Key to its goals is the building up of capacity and research skills, and for midwives and nurses this will mean enhancing their ability to understand, critique and proficiently utilize research in their respective fields of practice. Research in this context has particular meaning. The A-level notion of a library-based activity of collecting secondary information on a topic of interest will not suffice. Rather it is seen as a systematic inquiry that uses disciplined methods to answer questions or solve

**Table 7.1** Hierarchy of evidence

| Category level | Title | Description |
|---|---|---|
| I | Meta-analysis | A statistical analysis that combines or integrates the results of several independent clinical trials following a systematic review of the literature |
| II | Randomized controlled trial | A single well-designed RCT using powerful inferential statistics testing hypotheses predicting the impact of independent variables |
| | | The researcher introduces manipulation and measures for an effect (dependent variable) |
| III | Non-randomized trial | An experimental study involving hypothesis testing but less rigorous than an RCT since subjects cannot be randomly assigned to the control or experimental groups for some legitimate reason |
| IV | Non-experimental studies | Well-designed survey which may uncover a correlation or association between variables but unable to determine cause and effect relationships |
| V | Descriptive studies | Those studies, possibly excluding those of a qualitative nature, which provide accurate descriptive accounts of phenomena of interest or merely report expert opinion |

(Adapted from Muir-Gray, 1997)

problems. 'The ultimate goal of research is to develop, refine, and expand a base of knowledge' (Polit-O'Hara and Beck, 2006:4).

It is important for students to note the source and characteristics of any definition since this indicates an underlying philosophy, which may support or reject approaches to research. In this example note the emphasis placed on the utility value of any endeavour that seeks to be known as research.

Research provides much of the strongest evidence to support and direct nursing and midwifery practice but students must recognize that there are various types of research and each type has its particular function. Types of research may be viewed as a toolbox or tray of surgical instruments. And whilst it has been known for a screwdriver handle to be used as a hammer this is not recommended! Just as an expensive diamond-tipped ophthalmic scalpel will be useless to a midwife performing an episiotomy, an 'experiment' is quite inappropriate to *describe* the experiences of clients with learning disabilities in their interactions with a GP or practice nurse.

# Classifications of research

Research is taught and learned within classification frameworks. Such a compartmentalization is useful to the beginner who may have to critically appraise published research or even write a research proposal for their course. The trainee chef will doubtless follow the recipe book to the letter before he can expect to graduate as a TV celebrity devising original dishes or doing away with junk food in schools. However, as you begin to grasp research related concepts you will be able to see beyond these frameworks and move on to undertake higher-level studies requiring critical evaluation of research.

Research may be classified by its main purpose, for example to test a hypothesis, or more commonly according to its design, for example survey or another type. These ways of classifying research are fully explained, but first several more traditional two-dimensional classification frameworks are outlined in Table 7.2. While in some cases a piece of research may not conform neatly to these categories it is generally possible to place research within each of these.

## 'Purpose' as a classification

These two-dimensional classifications may clarify our understanding of the concept research but an additional way of viewing research is to focus on the main purpose or task the research is intended to accomplish. Many students come to research studies with the very narrow view that research is solely about testing a hypothesis. Within the frameworks presented this type of research could be classified as primary, quantitative, applied and experimental. Reading research reports soon demonstrates however that many researchers do not intend to test a hypothesis.

Researchers may set out to simply describe something, a situation that is not fully understood where an accurate or very detailed account is required.

*Descriptive research* may be employed to answer questions such as: 'How is informed consent obtained?' This may be directed to specific situations such as an unaccompanied child with acute injuries or an adult with learning disabilities requiring extensive dental work.

*Explanatory research* may follow on from a descriptive study or seek explanations for established facts. It may be well known that people who deliberately self-harm generally experience coolness or even hostility from general nursing and other staff when they present at a walk-in centre or accident and emergency department. A research study may simply set out to determine why this is, resulting in an accurate explanation of this common situation.

*Evaluation research* denotes the predetermined purpose and intention of the

**Table 7.2**  Research classification and description

**Classification and description**

**Pure research** is foundational research where the researcher may be curiosity-led, attempting cutting edge discoveries without practical applications in mind in advance. Utility value often comes to light but was not envisaged at the design stage. Associated with mathematics or the sciences. The older universities support this sort of research.

**Applied research** takes as its starting point a live question, hypothesis or problem and is intended to produce findings which have direct or indirect benefits. The newer universities, pharmaceutical industry and NHS Trust research departments will support this type of research.

**Primary research** is original work where the research collects data from subjects, e.g. clients or carers, attempting to add new knowledge to what is already known.

**Secondary research** is where information sources, e.g. completed research studies, are scrutinized and may be subject to a new analysis. Re-analysing large amounts of existing research provides the knowledge base to inform evidence-based practice. This approach may also be used in literature reviews which may demonstrate the need to conduct primary research.

**Quantitative research** has been characterized as being like the engineer searching for oil deposits. It starts with a detailed predetermined plan. The underlying philosophy reflects the scientific epistemology supporting the view that 'hard facts' amenable to measurement do exist. Quantification on numeric scales is the norm, e.g. Anxiety Score for clients receiving mental health nursing interventions. Physiological measurement or a highly structured questionnaire would each be described as quantitative. This is intrinsically linked with logical positivism.

**Qualitative research** is situated at the opposite end of a continuum from quantitative research. Characterized as exploratory, using unfolding designs seen as appropriate where the topic has not been researched very much and the subject defies quantification. This is intrinsically linked with naturalism and seeks in-depth holistic insights. The opposing concepts on these dimensions may be used to describe the research design, the data being collected, the method used to collect or analyse that data or even the researchers themselves.

**Experimental research** is a form of quantitative research embracing many complex designs including randomized controlled trials. Essentially it sets out to test predetermined variables to support or falsify a hypothesis which predicts a cause and effect relationship. A drug trial, sometimes using a placebo, is a typical example but 'experiment' is also used to investigate the effect of a given therapeutic approach.

**Non-experimental or observational** research has different purposes and designs from that of an experiment. This classification embraces many designs which set out to describe a number of variables. An essential distinguishing characteristic is that an observational study, unlike an experimental one, makes no attempt to manipulate any aspect of the phenomena under consideration.

researchers. This is its key distinguishing feature and in terms of design or methodology it is not restricted. Such a study may be classified as observational, primary and display both quantitative and qualitative elements. It may also follow the general pattern of a recognized design type such as a case study (discussed later). While there are models of evaluation research such as a needs-based evaluation or a cost–benefit evaluation (Robson, 2006) the term is essentially nothing more than a label to indicate its primary purpose.

*Practice improvement.* Most types of research may produce clear findings and be considered excellent quality when subjected to critical scrutiny. Even where a dissemination strategy has been carefully executed and there are unmistakable direct implications for practice it is possible, indeed quite probable, that much of this simply gathers dust inside journal covers. Yet the researchers may, by intention and design, desire to effect necessary improvements to practice. This purpose may require a multi-stage project incorporating research and change management in an integrated design. One such design is Action Research.

*Emancipatory or participatory research* is increasingly used with groups who may be relatively marginalized in society and have limited status or influence. Beyond this, such groups, for example people with enduring mental health problems, asylum seekers or more generally disabled people, may suffer stigma or discrimination even in their associations with midwifery or nursing services. Some researchers will set out to give voice to such groups via research and seek to involve participants at all stages of the research process even to the extent of devising the research aims. They may wish to simply place their research skills at the disposal of the given marginalized group (Northway, 2000).

*Consensus formation* may be the main purpose for other researchers or teams. They may wish to determine what a group of experts or key people think or predict about a service development in order for appropriate plans to be made. The purpose may then be to find a consensus among the carefully selected group. This sort of purpose may be absolutely in line with the needs of a senior management team within an NHS Primary Care Trust with responsibility for community-based services for older people or clients with learning disability. If a clear consensus among community matrons were known, staff training, skill mix and reshaping person specifications for new posts could all be put in place to support the changing demands of service users. A particular type of survey called a Delphi technique may provide the right tool in this case.

A common error students make in their attempts to critically evaluate published research is to misunderstand or neglect the main purpose of the research. Sometimes students judge all research as if it was engaged in hypothesis testing, disregarding the real purpose, which should be made clear by the aims or research question, often explicitly stated in the abstract.

# Research designs

There are numerous research designs that may be viewed as templates to use for a given research study. It is the main purpose of any given research project which should influence the design selected, which is a matter of using the correct tools for the task in hand. A research design is like the blueprint for a project connecting its driving aims, questions or hypotheses to the data which will be needed to achieve these ends, producing usable findings or results. Some designs are firmly fixed plans (pre-structured) whereas others develop as the research progresses (unfolding), a distinction eloquently described by Punch (2000).

The norms and conventions which characterize a recognized research design offer guidelines and structure to novice researchers and those who must critically appraise or critique research for use in practice or a specific academic module. However, while the textbooks and lecturers may suggest that these are mutually exclusive recipes for research, as different as cheese scones and granary bread, the reality is that the lines of demarcation are less clear. In fact one feature of some published research is that papers fail to explicitly identify with a specific design and students will have to deduce this for themselves by drawing out characteristics from the limited detail which is provided in a journal article. Within 'qualitative' research there is a tendency not to conform to a design template, perhaps using an eclectic approach and simply acknowledging the research as being qualitative.

Table 7.3 provides an overview of selected research designs which will help you appreciate the characteristics and appropriate utilization of a range of common research designs.

# Reviewing literature

There is clearly a need to discover the state of knowledge on a given topic as a key stage of the research process. This may be clearly demonstrated by performing a systematic search (see Chapter 6), obtaining, reading and reviewing studies. A literature review has been defined as the effective evaluation of selected documents (Hart, 1998).

While conducting a review of the literature has the potential to fulfil many functions, as part of the process of conducting research its primary function is to justify the need to conduct more primary research. To show that there is a gap in the knowledge and that the research topic is important are key to determining the necessity of proposed research. Establishing these two facts is increasingly seen as a pre-requisite for approval and, where appropriate, for funding applied

**Table 7.3** Overview of research designs

| Research design | Classification | Driving purposes | Key features |
|---|---|---|---|
| Experiment, quasi-experiment + randomized controlled trial | The terms primary, quantitative and experiment all fit this design<br><br>May be pure but in health care, usually applied | These designs set out to determine if there is a cause and effect relationship between variables of interest<br><br>Explanatory via hypothesis testing | Hypothesis and null hypothesis are devised.<br>Randomization of subject to experimental group – exposed to experimental conditions e.g. new drug<br><br>Control group may be exposed to a placebo or no manipulation at all<br><br>Measurement of variables e.g. physiological characteristics or stress scores |
| Survey | Usually primary but may be secondary<br><br>Commonly quantitative, non-experimental and applied | Quite versatile, may examine trends, knowledge or attitudes<br><br>May explore for possible correlation or simply describe things | Large numbers of participants, often uses questionnaire and relatively inexpensive<br><br>Usually attempts to generalize findings from sample to population<br><br>Many variations to consider e.g. cross sectional, longitudinal |
| Delphi survey technique | Quantitative, non-experimental, applied | Consensus formation; this sets out to describe a consensus attempting to predict future trends | Postal or e-mail contact with individual respondents<br><br>Identities kept secret to avoid influence<br><br>Several rounds where issues are identified, placed in rank order, analysed and re-presented to respondents in a series of contacts until a consensus is reached |
| Action research | Usually classified as qualitative but often mixed using quantitative data also<br><br>Applied and non-experimental, but may be viewed as an 'experiment in-situ' | Practice improvement<br><br>This design makes attempts to change, usually improve practice<br><br>Participatory or emancipatory goals may be explicit | This is usually a locally-based project<br><br>Team of stakeholders is established<br><br>Seeks wide involvement<br><br>Medium-term duration |

**Table 7.3** Continued

| Research design | Classification | Driving purposes | Key features |
|---|---|---|---|
| | | | Unfolding approach which may incorporate aspects of other recognized designs e.g. survey |
| | | | Issues or problems must be identified and carefully documented |
| | | | A plan is devised, changes implemented and evaluated |
| Case study | Qualitative but often mixed using quantitative data<br><br>Applied, primary and non-experimental | Descriptive, may introduce a comparative element<br><br>May be emancipatory or participatory | The researchers define the 'case' for this type of research study<br><br>Data triangulation employed to ensure detailed comprehensive description of the setting<br><br>Employs multiple methods of data collection, very flexible unfolding design which may leave no stone unturned |
| Historical | Not usually referred to as 'pure' but often curiosity-led<br><br>May be applied in the sense of shedding light on the present in explaining its historical context<br><br>May be primary or secondary depending on the availability of sources<br><br>Adopts a mixed approach drawing on both quantitative and qualitative data | Descriptive or explanatory | Chronology and context are vital<br><br>Aims to access primary sources whenever possible, these include hospital records, correspondence, diaries, minutes and papers from governing bodies<br><br>May be augmented by oral history<br><br>Highly flexible design |

(Continue overleaf)

| Design | Classification | Purpose | Features |
|---|---|---|---|
| Grounded theory | Qualitative, non-experimental, applied, primary | Explanatory explicitly in generating theory from data | Theoretical sampling and constant comparative method of analysis means that the processes of data collection and analysis are interactive<br><br>Emerged from sociology |
| Ethnography | Primary, qualitative, non-experimental, applied | Descriptive – very deep analytical description is desired<br><br>'Critical' ethnography seeks to change power relationships | Particular focus on culture or sub culture<br><br>May be large (macro) or small (micro) in scale<br><br>Participant observation is the key data collection method seeking an 'emic' or insider perspective<br><br>Prolonged engagement |
| Phenomenology | Primary, qualitative, non-experimental, applied | Descriptive interpretations of the reality of others<br><br>May incorporate an emancipatory or participatory goal | Seeks insights with applications to other settings<br><br>Purposive sampling to ensure that participants have experience in the area of interest e.g. fatigue associated with MS<br><br>Subjective 'lived experiences' and meaningfulness to respondents are investigated<br><br>Researchers use a technique known as bracketing in an attempt to suspend their own preconceived ideas<br><br>Uses in-depth interview to see the world from the clients' point of view |

N.B. Most of these designs do not feature on the hierarchy of evidence and some research papers do not neatly conform to any template design.

research (Scullion, 2000; Department of Health, 2006a). Performing a literature review is therefore essential and is conducted, with few exceptions, prior to commencement of a research project.

Your course will require you to be able to evaluate the quality of a literature review as part of published research papers and within a higher degree you will need to justify your own research, largely on the basis of your literature review. However, diploma or first-degree courses will inevitably involve students in carrying out literature reviews as a stand-alone academic exercise. You may have considerable choice in selecting a topic of interest but irrespective of this the skill, processes and discipline involved will be transferable to professional practice whenever you are faced with a knowledge deficit. Where there is a considerable amount of research the need for further research is questionable. A systemic review of the literature may provide clear direction to practice or provide robust answers to questions that have arisen from practice. See Box 7.1.

The NHS set up the Centre for Reviews and Dissemination in 1994, which freely offers rigorous and systematic reviews of research on selected topics. Based at the University of York (2006) it aims to provide research-based information about the effects of interventions used in health and social care and thus promotes the use of research-based knowledge. Students will find their website and publications invaluable.

## Stages in conducting a literature review

- Define the scope of the review – where the exercise is not undertaken as part of the research process it may be more clearly directed if a clear overall aim or even driving question is devised

---

**Box 7.1**   Characteristics of a good literature review

A literature review is not just a summary, but a conceptually organized synthesis of the evidence included. It should:

- Organize information and relate it to the research questions or aims of the review
- Clearly acknowledge the strength of the body of evidence
- Synthesize results into a summary of what is and isn't known
- Identify controversy when it appears in the literature
- Analyse the implications of the findings which may support or challenge current practice in midwifery or nursing
- Develop questions for further research.

---

- Identify the sources of relevant information – this is embodied in the 'search strategy' and is supported by explicit inclusion/exclusion criteria
- Review the literature – effective evaluation requires a good grasp of research concepts, an ability to identify the nature of the evidence and skill in critiquing research of various types
- Write the review – while most researchers and students would structure this according to emerging, not predetermined, themes it may be more appropriate to follow a chronological approach. Others may choose to divide it into literature of a theoretical nature followed by an examination of empirical literature based on research in which findings are presented. (Based on Carnwell and Daly, 2001.)

# Critiquing research

As a student you are seeking your first or additional qualification in midwifery or one of the many branches of nursing. Unless your course is a higher degree at masters or PhD level you are not studying to become a researcher. However, critiquing research is something that all nurses and midwives should be able to do in relation to their own field of practice and students will doubtless be assessed on their ability to do so. This skilled activity has become essential for all health professionals, aptly illustrated by Cutcliffe and Ward (2003:14) who warn that:

> If practitioners remain relatively unskilled in critiquing research, it is possible to implement evidence that is not only poor in quality and unrepresentative of that available, but it may have detrimental effects when inappropriately implemented into practice.

Rees (1997:31) writing primarily about midwifery research defines a critique as 'a careful consideration of both the strengths and limitations of published research'. Cutcliffe and Ward (2003:10) whose book provides several models for critiquing research and focuses primarily on mental health describes the process as 'reading an article, manuscript or paper, in a critical manner, in order to gauge the quality of the research'. Irrespective of your discipline each of these will prove invaluable to a student who is required to produce a critique of a piece of research.

Critiquing research has been conceptualized by Brink and Wood (1988:59) as 'a simple matter of asking a series of questions'. And many of the published guides present such questions which can be used to interrogate a given piece of research to enable you to draw conclusions about its nature, strength and quality. Yet these guides may themselves be based on assumptions and one common assumption is that all research is quantitative in nature. If such a guide were used to evaluate qualitative research such as a 'grounded theory' study you will conclude that it is very poor indeed unless you realize that the tool is not suitable for the task. One of your first considerations therefore is to ensure that the 'series of questions' you use is an appropriate one and even then published guides often neglect some key issues as highlighted by Cutcliffe and Ward (2003):

- Accessibility to target users – if the key people who need to be influenced by the findings are budget holders, is it known that this group of people actually read the journal where the research in question was published?
- Impact (or potential) on practice – this may be direct, indirect or methodological when the tools used in the research, rather than the findings, may be useful to your practice setting
- Key points for practice – to what extent does the research report specify how practice should change and are the recommendations feasible?
- Benefits to you, the reader – has the research developed your own understanding of the process, e.g. use of statistics, or challenged you to reflect on aspects of your practice or even your attitudes?

## Guidelines for critiquing research

Many of the things you have considered in this chapter are pertinent to the intellectual activity of appraising the quality of a research paper and inevitably there will be some repetition in the following guidelines. This activity is favoured by course directors and often features in mandatory modules at both CPD and pre-registration levels as part of the assessment strategy. Students will be given a research report, or may be asked to make their own selection, and required to submit a research critique based on this.

In keeping with the need for an appropriate 'series of questions' we include a generic list of questions and pointers complemented by additional comments concerning quantitative and qualitative research respectively.

After reading the paper questioningly, each of the following should be considered in relation to the research paper you are critiquing:

- Ensure you have a firm grasp of the detail of the paper so that you can describe it accurately
- Explore in detail the particular design used, e.g. case study or survey. This will mean reading a chapter or book devoted to this topic and considering the extent to which the norms of the design are evident in the research paper. Where there is a departure, is this justifiable?
- Consider whether a knowledge gap has been identified. Is this research both important and necessary?

- Examine the driving aim, research question or hypothesis. Are they supported by the literature review?
- Is there consistency between the aim, question or hypothesis, the data collection and analysis methods and the design selected? Review Tables 7.3 and 7.4 to assist you to determine which designs may be appropriate
- Has the sampling technique been described and is this appropriate?
- Was appropriate ethical approval and monitoring in place? To what extent were the rights of participants upheld? Was an ethical code used to underpin the study?
- How was recruitment and data collection actually administered and would these processes add or detract from the overall quality of the data obtained?
- Is there evidence of triangulation and if so was it used to good effect?
- To what extent are the findings presented linked to the actual data? Is it comprehensive or have certain points been emphasized? In qualitative data, are the themes adequately illustrated? Where verbatim quotes from respondents are used how have they been selected for inclusion?
- Do the findings match the researcher's interpretation of these, often covered under the heading 'discussion'? Are there alternative explanations?
- Are any implications for practice specified, which may be direct – new treatment superior to existing treatment; indirect – provides a trigger to reflect or enhance insights, e.g. the experience of fatigue in MS; methodological – instruments or processes used, rather than the findings, may be useful in clinical practice
- Are recommendations justified by the findings and presented in user-friendly ways?
- Have limitations been acknowledged and could any of these have been avoided or designed out? Were any lessons from the literature learned?
- Be aware of the constraints of the journal or other medium where the research was published. Check the 'author contributors guide' to assist here.

# Issues pertaining to quantitative research

### Validity

This is a multi-faceted concept that in essence is concerned with the extent to which research truly measures what it set out to measure and how truthful the research results are. However, the concept being measured may not lend itself to direct measurement. A fairly abstract concept such as 'hope' requires a valid indicator which indirectly but convincingly taps into this concept.

**Table 7.4** Essential concepts in critiquing research designs

| Research design | Essential concepts and issues |
| --- | --- |
| Experiment, quasi-experiment + randomized controlled trial | Selection criteria<br>Independent variable/s<br>Dependent variable/s<br>Ethical concerns, equipoise, subject understanding of randomization<br>Extraneous variables<br>Inferential statistics and probability (P-value) |
| Survey | Population<br>Relies on self-reporting<br>Validity, reliability, sampling technique<br>Representativeness and generalizability<br>Descriptive or inferential statistics used<br>The term 'survey' is used by some to mean 'questionnaire' |
| Delphi survey technique | Identification of 'experts'<br>Expert views expressed to form the consensus may themselves be uninformed about the latest research findings<br>Status of expert opinion |
| Action research | Particular ethical dilemmas concerning consent<br>Ownership<br>Key personnel and their ability to sustain any changes introduced<br>Similarity with audit |
| Case study | Transferability of findings to other settings<br>Beware of the potential to confuse this with 'care study' which examines the care of one patient |
| Historical | 'Presentism': tendency to view the past through the blurred lens of the present<br>May be linked to history of medicine<br>Consider why data sources were originally collected |
| Grounded theory | Role of literature review is debated<br>Saturation<br>Viewed as simply a data analysis technique by some<br>Experience of researcher may impact on quality as this is seen as a difficult approach |
| Ethnography | Extent to which researchers were immersed in the setting<br>Member checking or respondent validation |
| Phenomenology | Transferability of insights to novel settings<br>'Life-world'<br>Links with 'discovery interviews' in patient care<br>Literature review and researcher's preconceived ideas<br>Possibility of involvement of people who are relatively inarticulate |

More generally the validity of a study refers to the extent to which it relates to the topic and setting of the study without being unduly hindered by flaws in the design or processes.

## Reliability

This is the extent to which a measurement tool (for example a questionnaire or blood test) can be relied upon to provide results which are consistent over time, assuming the concept being measured has not itself altered. If the tool is reliable then replication of the study would produce similar results over time or where the measurement is carried out by different researchers. Reliability may be improved where the instruments are well established, used appropriately and supported by specific statistical tests. Macnee and McCabe (2008) elaborate on this and related concepts in their chapter on data collection methods.

## Statistics

Numeric data and its analysis are central to quantitative research.

- Do the statistics presented provide a clear descriptive summary of groups of data?
- Where inferential statistical tests are employed have the results reached statistical significance? A 'P' value of 0.05 or less usually determines this.
- Are these explicitly linked to the original hypotheses?
- Where group differences are established how significant is this to clinical practice?

# Issues pertaining to qualitative research

## Trustworthiness

This refers to the extent to which the whole research appears to be credible, including the researcher's credentials. The results should be considered in relation to dependability, confirmability, free from the researcher's biases and prejudices. Much of this can be determined by examining the processes employed at each stage of the research, in particular evidence of robust respondent validation whereby initial result of data analysis are returned to original informants for their approval or correction.

## Transferability

Transferability refers to how applicable the research findings are to another setting. The readers are left with these decisions but sufficient detail of the original setting is necessary to facilitate this judgement.

## Focus on design

Where the research specifies the design used or you can detect characteristics in the paper which are in keeping with a particular design you should give some emphasis to relevant essential concepts and issues. Table 7.4 highlights many of these and while some of the terminology may be unfamiliar you should explore these in more depth as an important part of the critique.

In addition to these pointers, where undertaken for a course or module requirement the university will provide some specific direction for the assignment. You may be required to give emphasis to the context of research in your particular field of practice or pay special attention to appraising the ethical aspects of the study. It is essential that you deal with this by:

1  Making sure you understand the scope and nature of the task
2  Reviewing the module outcomes
3  Planning to address every detail
4  Checking that you have addressed every detail prior to submission.

In view of the tendency to employ mixed research designs the application of guides to critiquing which focus on both quantitative and qualitative research may be required. In summary the key goals of a research critique can be achieved by interrogating research with the following questions:

- What is this?
- Can it be trusted?
- Is it applicable to my client group or me?

Qualities of a good critique are outlined below:

- Balanced – negative and positive points
- Constructive and unbiased
- Uncovers what lies behind the research
- Reflection on the whole research process
- Comprehensive even where the report appears to neglect issues, typically ethical considerations
- Provides a decisive analysis

- Avoids simply describing the research process
- Points made are supported by evidence and logically argued
- Makes recommendations
- Shows the extent to which findings may or should influence practice.

## Conclusions

Proficient use of evidence, mainly derived from research sources, is in effect a professional and ethical obligation to support clients and patients through nursing or midwifery interventions. It is vital that students and everyone on the professional register develop sufficient knowledge and skill in making judgements about the nature and strength of evidence and one of the ways in which this is achieved is through critiquing research. Only a few midwives or nurses will become researchers but increasing numbers are engaging in higher degrees which involve undertaking research. For the majority of students however the pressing task is the proficient use of research to justify or challenge practice or associated guidelines. The rationale for practice which once amounted to reliance on an authority embodied in the well-worn phrase 'Sister says . . .', more recently replaced with its equivalent 'Research says . . .', needs to change. Blindly following the findings of research may amount to no more than hearsay whereas what is emerging is a professional workforce which maintains research awareness and that can weigh up the evidence and proficiently apply this to complex patient care situations.

# Part 4

Demonstrating proficiency through assessment

# 8

# Critical analysis and higher-level skills for nurses and midwives

*Introduction • Skills and attributes • The need for critical analysis • Related concepts • Critical thinking • Developing critical analysis • Problem solving • Conclusion*

This chapter illustrates the need for critical analysis in the context of other skills and attributes necessary for nursing and midwifery. Levels of 'cognitive' skills are examined using a well-established hierarchy, which has considerable influence on nursing and midwifery education. It explains the concepts related to critical analysis and provides exercises designed to help you understand and develop associated higher-level skills. It provides a framework that will assist in developing analysis and critical evaluation with a worked example and related exercise. These topics are very relevant to the theory behind many assessments and this is briefly alluded to; however, this chapter provides a foundation of understanding which will help you to engage with the following chapter on assessment. Problem solving, an activity vital for nursing and midwifery requiring the use of critical analysis and higher-level skills, is also covered.

# Introduction

The term 'critical analysis' may seem scary to some nurses and midwives. Those who have been qualified for a decade or longer may feel this is too analytical and 'academic' for them. Undergraduate midwifery and nursing students may feel that to be critical is alien to their view of the 'caring' nature of their chosen profession and the imperative to be non-judgmental. Each are understandable starting points yet they probably reflect a limited understanding of the concepts involved since Quinn (2000:79), a very experienced teacher and author on nurse education, asserts that 'critical thinking is very different from criticism, in that it is basically a positive activity'. Far from being an academic concept of relevance only to essay writing and related activities, the 'demonstration of critical thinking in the clinical setting is a universally expected behaviour' (Mangena and Chabeli, 2005:292). Martin (1996:8) claims that unless we develop critical analysis and higher-level skills we will 'continue to accept care decisions without question', which would seriously undermine the need for evidence-based practice. Within assessments and university courses critical analysis is clearly a skills set which is an essential and explicit requirement. However, two decades after the then UK governing body (UKCC, 1986) proposed that a nurse should be an autonomous 'knowledgeable doer' this remains a central goal in nursing and midwifery education. These knowledge-based higher-level skills are very relevant when writing an essay and in assessments but primarily they are required to underpin clinical practice at all levels from newly qualified to specialist or consultant.

# Skills and attributes

Nursing and midwifery are often viewed as largely practice-based professions. However, the skills set required for any given branch or level within nursing or midwifery is broad and there is likely to be a commonality across disciplinary boundaries.

### Exercise 8.1

This exercise could be usefully carried out in a group with representatives from different branches of nursing and midwifery or even an interdisciplinary group. It could also be effectively undertaken alone in the isolation of your place of study.

- Spend some time thinking about what you do as a nurse or midwife or what your future role entails
- Make a rapid but extensive list of skills and attributes required to carry out these roles proficiently
- It may help to take one specific example related to a client and identify the required skills and attributes, select one from your own experience or Box 8.1
- Now try to place these skills and attributes into groups that share characteristics, e.g. are they mainly practical skills or are the emotional elements prominent?
- Where you are working with others, discuss the similarities and differences in the skills and attributes and how you have grouped them

You may have found that you classified the skills and attributes by their practical nature, their interpersonal nature, or even the underpinning knowledge. A common classification is to consider attributes within the following domains of learning:

- psychomotor
- affective
- cognitive.

## Psychomotor

The psychomotor domain includes physical movement, manipulative skills, manual dexterity, coordination, and the development of motor skills. Development of these skills requires practice, supervision and feedback. It is concerned with the execution of a skilled performance that underpins the practice base

---

**Box 8.1**  Patient related examples – identify the required attributes and skills

- Dealing with a mother and family where a stillbirth has occurred
- An aggressive informal in-patient on a psychiatric assessment unit who wishes to leave the hospital
- An unconscious 9-year-old child who has sustained lacerations following what may have been a seizure
- A teenage girl with seriously reduced capacity in her urinary bladder who is upset by this
- A 48-year-old man following treatment for myocardial infarction, almost ready for discharge

---

of midwifery and nursing. Psychomotor skills are developed and assessed on practice placements and in university-based skills laboratories.

## Affective

In psychology the term 'affect' is used to describe a person's externally displayed mood. The affective domain includes feelings, values, appreciation, enthusiasm and motivation. It is concerned with the entire spectrum of values and value systems. It concentrates on emotions and attitudes associated with both processes and outcomes of learning. It is particularly relevant to the caring professions, e.g. the art of nursing, but is relatively neglected in formal study.

## Cognitive

The cognitive domain of learning is concerned with the development of intellectual abilities and skills. It equates with the 'science' components of the professions and concerns processing information, 'cognition' or thinking.

Look back at your list of professional skills and attributes and see if items you identified fit primarily into any of these three categories. While you will find that some skills or attributes are complex and have elements of all three, others will fit neatly into just one of these categories. Educators acknowledge that learning in all three areas involving skills, attitudes and knowledge is essential especially for complex professional roles such as nursing or midwifery. Much of what is taught and assessed and much of what you are required to learn can be traced back to these three domains of learning and even limited reading in this area will lead you to their historical origins in Bloom's taxonomies (Bloom, 2006). These are essentially classification systems and levels of learning for each of the three domains, psychomotor, affective and cognitive.

The cognitive taxonomy (Bloom, 2006) presents a hierarchy of levels of learning starting with knowledge at its base (see Table 8.1).

These cognitive levels inform learning objectives or outcomes which may be used to describe the intentions of educational events. These could include the whole course, a placement or module or even an individual seminar, lecture or practical skills session. If you examine the declared objectives or outcomes you will know what is required and these can then be used either to prepare for the experience (e.g. a placement or lecture), or check that your achievements are at the required level.

Undeniably nurses and midwives must possess specific practical skills such as airway maintenance and drug administration. They must also have attributes related to attitudes and values, emotional resilience, empathy and good interpersonal skills, which fall into the 'affective' domain. Yet these are interrelated and to a large extent dependent on 'cognition' or thought processes and the

Table 8.1 Hierarchy of cognitive levels from Bloom's taxonomy

| Knowledge | Comprehension | Application | Analysis | Synthesis | Evaluation |
|---|---|---|---|---|---|
| Ability to accurately bring to mind information and facts | Understanding facts, perhaps demonstrated by summarizing or explaining the information or facts in your own words | Utilization of knowledge, which is understood, into real situations Ability to apply rules, concepts or principles | Involves ability to break information into component parts, notice relationships among them and identify their relative importance | Ability to combine discrete information (components of your analysis) into a new kind of unique whole (e.g. a stance in an essay or a plan of action) | Making judgements regarding the value of something based on logical argument using appropriate evidence |
| | Builds on: knowledge | Builds on: knowledge + comprehension | Builds on: knowledge + comprehension + application | Builds on: knowledge + comprehension + application + analysis | Builds on: knowledge + comprehension + application + analysis + synthesis |

knowledge it generates: critical analysis and higher-level skills which are essentially cognitive. Together, progress in these domains of learning contributes to the 'knowledgeable doer' that you are, or aspire to be.

# The need for critical analysis

While knowledge and comprehension are vital, possessing these is relatively unimportant unless they are applied to midwifery or nursing situations. If a nurse had knowledge about the need for blood pressure monitoring following neuro-surgical procedures or closed head injury, along with the appropriate psycho-motor skills, she could undertake this practical skill knowledgeably and accurately and make the necessary records. If she failed to comprehend its significance or did not apply this knowledge to the specific patient then clearly there is a limitation in her cognitive level. Her cognitive level was clearly not sufficient for safe patient care as she failed to demonstrate both comprehension and application. However, higher-level cognitive abilities enabling you to assess and judge (analysis, synthesis and evaluation) are increasingly valued in health care environments, where all health care practitioners are expected to base their practice on the best available evidence, according to Castle (2006), who is engaged in research on higher-level skills.

Fullerton and Thompson (2005) claim that for midwifery practice, critical thinking is an essential component of evidence-based practice. In the case of mental health nursing, Crowe and O'Malley (2006) claim that critical reflection skills are required for practitioners to be able to analyse and improve practice, particularly for advanced practice. They go on to provide some specific learning activities aimed at promoting critical thinking skills.

A natural development of critical analysis may be to gain insights into the political context of health care and the social determinants of health. This leads some nurses and midwives to challenge social and political factors, which contribute to the situation of many of their clients. The learning disability nurse may so identify with the stigma and discrimination faced by their client group that their own critical analysis leads them to a personal commitment to client advocacy. They may actively support pressure groups aimed at challenging and improving such circumstances.

Critical analysis is something qualified nurses and midwives do on a daily basis in their clinical practice. Demonstrating this in academic assignments however is often a different matter with students at all levels expressing difficulties, according to Gopee (2002), a prolific writer on educational issues. Assignment work frequently attracts comments from academic staff which suggest that work is too descriptive and the amount or depth of analysis or evaluation is insufficient. Weak essays and other academic assignments will often attract feedback such as:

- 'Generally descriptive in nature'
- 'Evidence is accepted uncritically'
- 'While you show a good level of knowledge there is little by way of analysis or evaluation'
- 'Tentative analysis is embryonic and needs to be developed'.

Clearly nurses and midwives need to develop their ability to critically analyse for many reasons, including crucially:

- to meet Nursing and Midwifery Council standards
- to justify practice and underpin skills
- commensurate with developing specialist and advanced roles
- to challenge ideas, both their own and in society more generally
- to address educational requirements set at predetermined academic levels
- to support professional attitudes.

Critical analysis is also important in enhancing:

- ability to act as patient/client advocate
- practice – linked to evidence-based practice
- problem-solving skills
- contribution by nurses and midwives to the inter-professional agenda.

# Related concepts

Terminology is often used imprecisely so it is worth pausing at this point to review and clarify terms used so far:

- From an analysis of its root, Castle (2003:369) points out that 'critical' implies making judgements 'based on values gained through evidence and is used in the questioning, investigative sense rather than the disapproving or fault-finding sense'
- 'Analysis' means the ability to break content into its components in order to identify parts, see relationships among them, and recognize organizational principles
- In academic terms 'critical analysis' implies 'considering the claims of theorists,

governments, authorities and so on, what they are based on, and how far they seem to apply or be relevant to a given situation' (University of Sussex, N.D.).

In some of the literature and perhaps in your course literature you will come across many related terms which are at times used interchangeably. They will be particularly prominent in information related to the assessments you will need to undertake.

You will see from Table 8.1 that within the cognitive domain terms related to levels of learning are defined but this hierarchy will sometimes be modified. Notice in particular that the concept 'critical' is missing from this hierarchy yet it is commonly used, especially in relation to the level of analysis or above. The term is liberally inserted into academic papers and module guides and is either implying an additional dimension, for example 'analysis +' or a device to make the requirement for rational examination of ideas explicit.

- **Critique** – often used in association with research, defined by Rees (1997:31) as 'a careful consideration of both the strengths and limitations'. This implies evaluation and all the cognitive attributes, which it builds on
- **Critical reflection** – has been defined as 'deliberately thinking or mulling over experiences with the intention of learning' (see Chapter 5). The term 'critical' suggests probing questions will be explored focusing on the rational application of evidence to the process
- **Critical evaluation** – at the lower levels such as knowledge, some students will describe things and uncritically accept and use evidence. However critical evaluation is used to give emphasis to the quality of logical argument that is actually integral to evaluation

It is important to read course materials which refer to these sorts of concepts and check with lecturers that you share a common understanding, especially as they are often used to describe the level of achievement you are required to meet. This will be particularly important when considering academic levels 1 to 3 and vital when you move between these levels, such as at the beginning of year three in your course.

# Critical thinking

Critical thinking is seen as a purposeful process involving arguments, assumptions, beliefs or actions making use of higher-level cognitive skills. The process involves interpretation of information, analysis, drawing conclusions and evaluation that may lead to challenging ideas or practices. In order to develop or demonstrate higher-level cognitive skills you must engage in critical thinking. Whilst in the past this was actively discouraged it is now seen as essential. Table 8.2, which is adapted from Scheffer and Rubenfeld (2000) and Castle (2006), outlines the components of critical thinking, the skills required and examples which demonstrate achievement of each component.

# Developing critical analysis

Like playing a musical instrument, some argue that you can only develop critical analysis, synthesis, evaluation and critical thinking, by actually doing it. There is therefore a need for practice and feedback, preferably before it arrives in the form of comments on an academic assignment, although this feedback should be viewed as essential for learning.

Gopee (2002) devised an excellent seven-stage framework, based on Bloom's cognitive taxonomy, which illustrates essential activities leading up to critical analysis.

This framework (see Table 8.3) will be useful in developing your own ability to critically analyse and also constitutes a useful checklist that may be used to judge progress in drafting an academic assignment.

It is obvious that 'students who wish to attain a clear pass in their assignments need to comprehend fully the appropriate criteria' (Gopee, 2002:47). Table 9.1 (in Chapter 9), gives an example of criteria that may be used to assess written assignments. It will be observed that this too can be traced back to its origins within a cognitive hierarchy, as is the case for most assessment criteria. Notice that academic levels roughly equate with years in a three-year course:

- Level (year) one – focuses on accurate understanding, this requires adequate knowledge and comprehension
- Level (year) two – expects utilization (application) of knowledge and analysis
- Level (year) three – integration and synthesis are required along with evaluation in addition to the lower-level cognitive skills.

### Exercise 8.2

- Obtain assessment criteria related to your course or module (often found in the student handbook)
- Map these criteria against cognitive levels
- Take a draft assignment or one you have had returned (e.g. essay)

**Table 8.2** Critical thinking skills

| Component | Skills required | Skill attainment (examples) |
|---|---|---|
| Information seeking | Seeker of knowledge, truth and understanding<br>Identify and search relevant sources for evidence or data | Able to search literature |
| Analysis | Divide the whole into parts to investigate the components, functions and relationships<br>Value focused, systematic and comprehensive approach to issues | Consider inequalities in health |
| Evaluation | Read the evidence and clarify issues<br>Assess accuracy and reliability<br>Make judgements and draw conclusions based on evidence | Assess a journal article or statistical dataset |
| Reflection | Consideration of past experiences or events to deepen understanding | Write a reflective diary |
| Creativity | Conceive, ascertain or review ideas to develop alternatives | Design a health promotion programme in clinical practice |
| Prediction | Envisage potential outcomes or consequences | Evaluate a case study |
| Discrimination | Differentiate between relevant and irrelevant<br>Identify inconsistencies<br>Recognize differences and similarities | Compare and contrast two approaches to behaviour modification or two similar journal articles |
| Context | Consider the background and influences relevant to an issue | Examine an issue within the context of a government policy |
| Perseverance | Use determination to overcome barriers or problems | Give an oral presentation |
| Flexibility | Able to adapt, modify or change thoughts in light of evidence | Patient assessment |
| Open-mindedness | Encompass divergent opinions<br>Address personal bias or prejudice | Address inequality or diversity issues |
| Knowledge transfer | Able to adapt and broadcast media to a specific audience | Produce patient education materials |
| Confidence | Become an effective communicator<br>Apply reasoning skills<br>Develop intuitive and insightful understanding | Give a presentation including a 'questions and answers' session<br>Academic viva voce |

**Table 8.3** Seven-stage framework of critical analysis (adapted from Gopee, 2002)

| | Stages | Cognitive levels |
|---|---|---|
| 1 | Identify and consider all the elements of the topic | Knowledge |
| 2 | Identify and select relevant information and knowledge | Knowledge and comprehension |
| 3 | Examine elements and knowledge to establish the relationships between different elements | Comprehension |
| 4 | Determine the context in which the topic is being examined | Application |
| 5 | Identify and then challenge assumptions or evidence for accuracy and validity in context | Application and analysis |
| 6 | Reflect, explore and imagine alternatives | Analysis |
| 7 | Draw justifiable conclusions about the topic being considered | Synthesis |

**Table 8.4** Nine-factor framework to develop critical evaluation

| | Factor |
|---|---|
| 1 | Identify and consider all elements of the selected topic |
| 2 | Select information and knowledge which is most relevant to the topic |
| 3 | Examine elements and knowledge to establish relationships between different elements |
| 4 | Determine the context in which the topic is being examined |
| 5 | Identify and then challenge assumptions and evidence for accuracy and validity in context |
| 6 | Reflect and imagine alternatives |
| 7 | Decide on your position by drawing justifiable conclusions about the topic being considered |
| 8 | Suggest a new approach to this topic or how things should be viewed, changed or challenged |
| 9 | Argue the value of this new approach or your suggestions |

- ○ Apply Gopee's seven-stage framework to determine what level of cognitive ability is being demonstrated
- ○ Use this as the basis for a tutorial

Gopee's (2002) framework for critical analysis has been adapted and extended to a nine-factor framework to assist in the development of critical evaluation. See Table 8.4.

Taking the general topic of 'disability' related to nursing and midwifery this framework could be used to develop all the higher-level cognitive skills, up to critical evaluation, as follows:

*Factor one*

- Classifications of disability (e.g. congenital or acquired)
- Objective measurement (e.g. DALYS, Barthel Index)
- Images of disabled people (i.e. wheelchair, children in need, charity)
- Legal protections against discrimination (e.g. Special Educational Needs and Disability Act 2001, Disability Discrimination Act 2005)
- Range of proposed causes of disability
- Role of health care professionals
- Disabled people's experiences of health, illness and health care services
- Range of terminology used and the 'politically correct' imperative

*Factor two*

- Legal protections against discrimination
- Proposed causes of disability; linked to models devised to explain the concept 'disability'
- Role of health care professionals, especially nurses and midwives
- Disabled people's experiences of health, illness and health care services
- Possible discrimination

*Factor three*

- Debate and argument over root causes of disability linked to models of disability, e.g. medical or social model
- Discrimination – examine links with other forms of discrimination, e.g. race, and consider the impact of models of disability and the experiences of disabled people as consumers of health care services
- Examine the legal requirements of service providers and their impact on the NHS

*Factor four*

- Current NHS policy related to public and patient involvement
- Disability related legal requirements on NHS
- Professional obligations
- Inequitable delivery of health care related to the status of clients as 'disabled people'

*Factor five*

- Assumptions linked to models
- Medical causes or social causes – often presented as diametrically opposite

- Medical: individual problems requiring individual adjustments or medical solutions
- Social: problems stem from society and medicine is deemed to be most blameworthy
- Examine the nature of the evidence (research) and its underlying assumptions (paradigms)

## Factor six

- How have I dealt with disabled people as clients or in general? (Personal and professional experiences.)
- Do the proposed models account for these experiences comprehensively?
- If medicine as an institution and, by association, midwifery and nursing are implicated as part of the problem what role, if any, does this leave for health professionals in the lives of disabled people?
- Does the truth lie somewhere between the two main extremes?

## Factor seven

- Disabled people experience what amounts to discrimination in many ways:
  - lower priority for health screening
  - limited accessibility to mainstream health services
  - negative values and disability related attitudes impact on medical decision making
  - many disabled people fear contact with health services
- There is sufficient evidence to implicate medicine as an institution (or medicalized ideas) as contributing to disability discrimination
- The majority of nurses and midwives subscribe to a medicalized notion of 'disability'
- There is a role for nurses and midwives in the lives of disabled people, e.g. in rehabilitation, during pregnancy etc. and illness unrelated to the disabled identity

## Factor eight

- Disability should be viewed as an equality issue by nurses and midwives and health services providers in general
- Negative views of disability within the professions should be challenged, e.g. via disability equality training
- Legal and policy obligations should be monitored
- Positive attempts should be made to involve disabled people as follows:
  - to audit the services provided by nurses and midwives

- ○ education at all levels, direct and indirect impact on curricula and training
- ○ employment/redeployment of disabled people (nurses, midwives and other health professionals) within the health services

### Factor nine

- This promotes equality, rights of disabled people as citizens, consumers and employees
- Social justice of this case
- Value disabled people as experts in consultations with health professionals
- Partnership, public and patient involvement
- Value of both medical and social models of disability

The above has taken the general topic of 'disability' and provided an example where this framework has been applied in the development of higher-level cognitive abilities. It will of course be the result of much discussion, critical thinking and reflection. A considerable amount of reading will also be required and, to complement the example above, Box 8.2 provides a brief bibliography. Although this has been quite general you may wish to reflect on its relevance to your own field of practice. With around 9 million disabled people in the UK there are implications for midwifery and all branches of nursing practice.

It is important however that you select a topic of your own choosing and work through these factors for yourself, and the following exercise will assist in this process.

### Exercise 8.3

Take a topic that you have a serious interest in, preferably one related to a forthcoming assignment. If this proves problematic, consider using one of the suggested topics listed below:

- breastfeeding among lower income mothers
- health implications for children following parental breakdown
- legal and media images of mental illness and their influences on community care
- social integration of people with learning disabilities – health care, employment, leisure
- pain management – from traumatic injury to rehabilitation and beyond
- amalgamating existing services as part of organizational restructuring.

N.B. Each of these may be modified by adding 'the role of the . . .' or 'implications for the . . .' midwife, child nurse, modern matron etc.

---

**Box 8.2**

Albrecht, G.L., Seelman, K.D., Bury, M. (eds) (2001) *Handbook of Disability Studies*. Thousand Oaks: Sage.

Bowling, A. (2005) *Measuring Health: A Review of Quality of Life Measurement Scales*, 3rd edn. Maidenhead: Open University Press.

Davies, S. (ed.) (2006) *Rehabilitation: The Use of Theories and Models in Practice*. Edinburgh: Churchill Livingstone.

Jones, B. (2003) *Childhood Disability in a Multicultural Society*. Abingdon: Radcliffe Medical Press.

Northway, R. (1997) Disability and oppression: some implications for nurses and nursing. *Journal of Advanced Nursing*, 26(4): 736–43.

Priestley, M. (1999) *Disability Politics and Community Care*. London: Jessica Kingsley.

Scullion, P. (2000) Disability as an equal opportunity issue within nurse education in the UK. *Nurse Education Today*, 20: 199–206.

---

- Using the nine-factor framework make brief notes of your current thoughts BEFORE undertaking any reading – concentrate on capturing your first thoughts
- After conducting a literature search and reading key sources think about this topic and if possible discuss your emerging thoughts with others
- Work through each of the nine factors and make notes related to each of them
- Compare your thoughts and conclusions after this exercise with the notes you made earlier which represented 'first thoughts' on the topic

This exercise will take considerable time to complete but not only will it assist in developing your ability to demonstrate higher-level cognitive skills, such as analysis, synthesis and evaluation, it may form an important part of the preparation for an assignment for your current course.

# Problem solving

Qualified nurses and midwives are faced daily with problems of various kinds and their chosen responses could have far-reaching effects. Students must develop competence and then proficiency in problem-solving skills particularly around the transition period from student to nurse or midwife. Professionally qualified practitioners must not just perform 'routine work and go off' (Mangena and Chabeli, 2005:297), rather education should produce 'practitioners who have the ability to identify, solve problems and make decisions through the use of critical and creative thinking', according to Mangena and Chabeli (2005:292), who strongly advocate critical thinking.

A study amongst midwifery and nursing students found that faced with a problem around a third avoided the problem and around a fifth did the first thing that came to mind! (Altun, 2003.) Less than half (97 out of 218 participants) attempted to solve the problem systematically, a process clearly requiring critical analysis and higher-level cognitive skills. The first thing when faced with a clinical or academic problem should in most circumstances, be the process of critical thinking.

### Exercise 8.4

- Review Table 8.1 and identify which components of critical thinking you have achieved
- Discuss these with a colleague (study buddy) and cite evidence to back up the claim that you have achieved these
- From those components where you recognize a need to develop, or other higher-level skills you need to improve on, devise an action plan to develop and demonstrate these skills – this may be something you could effectively do within a self-appointed study group

## Conclusion

Analysis, synthesis and evaluation are all cognitive skills that nurses and midwives need to use in their professional practice. Practising critical thinking and reflection will help you develop these higher-level skills. Debate, dialogue and discussion with colleagues, mentors and lecturers will all contribute to improving these abilities and enable you to grow in confidence and achievements in your attempts to demonstrate these skills in academic work and clinical practice.

# 9

# Coping with examinations and assessments

*Introduction • Value of assessment • Who assesses? • Formative or summative*
*• Practice-based assessment • Criteria • Preparing for success •*
*Cue-consciousness • Methods of assessment • Planning for success*
*in assessments • Characteristics of assessment methods • Plagiarism •*
*Difficult circumstances • Springboard to success • Conclusion*

This chapter briefly examines the justification, value and need for assessments and who assesses nurses and midwives. It distinguishes between formative and summative assessments and describes practice-based assessments. Assessment criteria are examined and an example is provided along with a related student feedback sheet.

Developing 'cue-sensitivity', a concept devised originally from research into how students cope with examinations (Miller and Parlett, 1974), will be encouraged to assist in the preparation for assessment and learning. Coping well with exams and other methods of assessment by effective preparation is linked to the specific circumstances making success more likely. Dealing with the disappointment of failure is not neglected and clear advice is offered on how to use this experience positively to ensure success at your second attempt and to transfer these skills to ensure you do well in other future assessments. The issue of plagiarism is examined. In relation to difficult circumstances which may hinder your performance in assessments, specific advice is offered.

# Introduction

I passed my driving test! But before you write out a congratulations card I must admit that it was my second attempt. Nevertheless I am authorized to drive and I have the licence to prove it. However, accident statistics, the proliferation of speed cameras and the rising cost of motor insurance, may indicate that drivers, most of whom have passed their test, do not always behave sensibly or legally. Likewise the standards of practice displayed by qualified nurses and midwives sometimes fall short of the NMC Code of Professional Conduct (Nursing and Midwifery Council, 2004a). Perhaps assessments, tests, exams and character references do not always accurately predict future behaviour, knowledge or good attitudes. But the fact remains that students of nursing and midwifery, whether pre-registration or CPD, will be assessed. There have been some concerns that nursing and midwifery courses have not fully prepared individuals for professional practice, particularly at pre-registration level (UKCC, 1999). The public and employers need to have confidence that qualifications reliably reflect a standard of knowledge and competence and this has given rise to an increased focus on assessment strategies. And while it must be acknowledged that assessment systems are imperfect they act as 'gatekeeper' to the professions and have a prominent place in the experience of students at all levels. You can learn to cope well with the various forms of assessment and by design or as a side effect you will learn a tremendous amount because of the assessments you must pass (Tang, 1994).

# Value of assessment

Some students take the view that if it is not assessed then it does not count and in one sense they are right. Nursing and midwifery courses have been notoriously over-assessed; perhaps following this belief and the pervading commitment to high quality patient care, everything is seen as important.

You may have come across people who are brilliant in exams but within a week have forgotten everything and furthermore are hopeless at dealing with clients and their families. You are likely to be faced with few exams in numeracy or pharmacology for example, but the range of methods of assessment used is vast. This approach is useful in that if you generally do not excel in exams you may perform better in other types of assessment. Some forms of assessment capture different qualities and a broad strategy is more comprehensive. This variety is also seen as adding to the fairness of assessments (Race and Brown, 2001). Therefore, on completion of the course you will be fit for purpose as well as having the award of diploma, degree or module credits.

# Who assesses?

Perhaps surprisingly it is not only your lecturers or mentors who are involved in the assessment process. On some courses you will be assessed by your own peers (Welsh, 2006) which counts for as much as 30% of the overall marks, and there is a growing trend to incorporate aspects of self-assessment. This is very much in line with the professional commitment to self-regulation, promoting reflection and higher-order cognitive skills (Price, 2005). Self-assessment is considered one of the most important skills that students require for effective learning and for future professional development and lifelong learning (National Committee of Enquiry into Higher Education, 1997:8–12), supporting the philosophy promoting independent active adult learning.

There are also good arguments for allowing clients to have a role in assessment of student nurses or midwives and this is beginning to move beyond tokenism as part of the public and patient involvement agenda (Forrest *et al.*, 2000; Walters and Adams, 2002).

# Formative or summative

The primary purpose of assessments that are designated 'formative' is to provide students with fairly reliable information about how they are doing. And while any assessment where feedback is provided may be diagnostic, formative assessment is primarily diagnostic. It will not contribute towards the overall pass or fail on a module or course and is sometimes optional. Before you dismiss it as 'does not count', consider how valuable it is to know how you are progressing. In a university system which may be alien to you this opportunity is too good to be missed. Jump at the chance, especially at an early stage of the course.

Most assessments will be designated 'summative', and these do contribute to the pass/fail decision. If opportunities to practise assessments arise then take them! Not only does this motivate, it provides valuable focused revision and vital feedback. It also has the effect of reducing the fear of the unknown, reducing stress and allowing you to adapt your approach to preparation, making it even more effective. Your lecturers may be helpful if you approach them for advice on practising assessments. If opportunities are not offered, then, either alone or with friends on the same course, manufacture them. Try to ensure that as many elements of the real thing are reproduced for your practice session. In the case of an exam the characteristics you are trying to reproduce include:

- unseen questions – ensure you do not know in advance
- restrictions on what may be taken into an examination room
- strict time limit without interruptions
- style of writing and method of dealing with mistakes.

# Practice-based assessment

In general assessments are designed to discriminate between those who have abilities, skills or knowledge at a certain level, and those who do not. They are refined by the introduction of grades beyond a mere pass or fail. Most academic work is graded on a percentage scale and performance in practice placements is also increasingly awarded a grade. Marking grids indicate what the marker is going to focus on and an astute student should do the same.

You will be supported in practice by a variety of staff. Practice-based assessment requires verification of your achievements from designated clinically based staff. Your mentor will play a key role in assessing your achievement and some universities use triads, whereby three key people determine the grade in practice collaboratively. These are the mentor, the university lecturer and the student herself. There is some evidence that in self-assessment good students tend to underrate themselves and weaker students overrate themselves (Dochy *et al.*, 1999:334). In the case of triads you should attempt to objectively consider the evidence for your own assessment and discuss this with the other two key people.

# Criteria

Most marking of exams or coursework will be criterion based. This means that you are not in competition with your peers. Your work will be judged according to published standards, which equate with academic levels, roughly in line with years one, two and three (see Chapter 8). CPD students will only undertake work at levels 2 or 3 unless the course is at masters degree level where appropriate M-level criteria will be used.

You should have access to the marking criteria in advance and any feedback should be linked to this. What your university uses is likely to be detailed but will have some resemblance to Table 9.1 which provides criteria for levels 1–3 which includes only the extremes of a high pass and fail examples.

Some assessments have their own specific criteria but these will be available in advance and will be useful in directing your preparations.

Some universities use a marking system which allows a maximum of 90 points to be awarded for excellent work. Others use a percentage system, which theoretically at least allows for 100%. Yet it is curious that students' work which is innovative and extending knowledge may be awarded little more than 70% as if there were an unwritten ceiling at about 70%, above which lecturers dare not stray! This is an interesting phenomenon that may be debated in official arenas

**Table 9.1** Marking criteria

| Academic level | Very high pass | Below pass standard |
| --- | --- | --- |
| One | Accurate use of relevant material presented logically | Ambiguous with limited understanding of concepts and issues |
| | Clear understanding of issues and their relationships | There are inaccuracies and the relevance of much of the material is not clear |
| Two | Analysis and reflections are clearly demonstrated | Reflection and analysis are not evident |
| | Critical understanding of literature and research which is utilized to integrate theory and practice | Relevant research or literature is not used to effectively show the integration of theory and practice |
| | | Clear understanding is not demonstrated |
| Three | Ability to synthesize based on analysis and reflection is clearly evident | Mainly descriptive with some analysis but lacking synthesis and evaluation |
| | An abundance of relevant research is applied to evaluate and integrate theory and practice | Application of theory to practice is limited and there is little or no demonstration of higher-level cognitive skills |

## Literature review – STUDENT FEEDBACK SHEET

Searching the literature

There is evidence of considerable effort in outlining the search strategy and a key strength is your use of the grey literature. However, the links to the main focus of the review are not always clear either in this section or your introduction. Exclusion criteria, e.g. your decision to exclude surveys, was not justified and this approach is not comprehensive. The three areas you focused on did not reflect your very broad title of the review.

Critical Evaluation

Quite a good level of knowledge of research is demonstrated and you use this to illustrate the nature of the evidence included in the review. Some studies are however merely described and appear to be accepted uncritically while others are critiqued.

Synthesis

While you make mention of many implications for practice, links to the underlying evidence are not made explicit and the policy context is neglected. Ideas are not coherently linked together and there is no well-reasoned argument presented. A rather jumbled attempt, partly reflecting the focus of the review, which is quite vague.

Organization and structure

The main focus of this review would have been made clearer if you had devised a clear aim or question to drive your interrogation of the literature. Some restructuring would enhance the logical progression of ideas and link identified themes more clearly.

Presentation

The document looks professional and is presented to a high standard. Your use of English is very good and you adhere to the approved style of Harvard referencing very closely. Academic style of writing is demonstrated quite well. This is a strength but is limited compensation for weaknesses in other areas.

Additional comments

A fair overall attempt with strengths and weaknesses. Showing a good appreciation of some of the literature and ability to critique. You fail to appreciate the global picture and this would not be adequate to base practice on. Needed to be more clearly focused but I note the considerable effort and developing ability to deal with this kind of assignment.

FIGURE 9.1 Literature review student feedback sheet

such as student consultative councils; it may be that 75% represents excellence in your university.

Table 9.2 reproduces a marking grid provided in a module handbook. It relates to a 10,000 word review of research literature on a topic selected by the student as the sole assessment for a level 3 double module.

### Exercise 9.1

- Read the grid presented in Table 9.2 and write in your own words what you have to do in order to achieve more than 70%
- What additional details do you require to direct your learning for this assignment?
- Now read the fictitious student feedback sheet related to the same module (see Figure 9.1 opposite) and decide what range of marks you would expect this to be awarded within each section and as an overall mark
- Later compare this with Table 9.3
- Obtain a similar marking guide or published criterion from a piece of work you are going to be assessed on
- Go through the processes outlined in the first two steps above
- Use this as the basis for discussion with your peers and the relevant lecturers at an early stage of the work concerned

# Preparing for success

Ideally the assessment you are preparing for coincides with the necessary learning and so you are using time effectively. Since assessment strategies are designed to test the extent to which you have learned, the first advice is to concentrate on improving your efficiency as a learner. This may mean going back to previous chapters of this book and dealing with any deficits that become apparent.

However, when you are in a position to focus on the assessment it is important to consider the following questions as part of your preparation:

- What is the purpose and nature of the assessment?
- Is there an element of choice and is this known in advance?
- How important is this assessment in relation to other assessed elements of the course?

Table 9.2 Marking guide for a literature review

| Percentage | Searching the literature | Critical evaluation | Synthesis | Organization and structure | Presentation |
|---|---|---|---|---|---|
| 70 | Very clear justification of search strategy<br><br>Comprehensive<br><br>Explicit link to main focus of review<br><br>Could easily be replicated from detail provided | Very clear appreciation of the nature of the evidence included in the review<br><br>Advanced research critiquing skills demonstrated<br><br>Evidence of analysis and application to the aim/question driving the review | Assembles and links concepts, theories and policy logically to build a strong well-reasoned argument clearly showing implications of the review for practice | A very clear area and focus for the review is identified<br><br>Clear, well-justified, coherent structure utilized to divide the work (chapters/themes) | Excellent use of English used accurately in an academic style<br><br>Layout is attractive and reader friendly<br><br>The Harvard system is used consistently facilitating ease in relocating all sources utilized |
| 60–69 | Search strategy justified fairly well<br><br>Comprehensive but leaves some key aspects unexplored<br><br>Links to main focus of review clear | Some of the evidence included is examined in relation to its nature and value<br><br>Critique of much of the literature is provided demonstrating very good knowledge of research | Assembles and links concepts, theories and policy logically<br><br>A well-reasoned argument is built showing implications of the review for practice | A clear area and focus for the review is identified<br><br>Coherent structure utilized to divide the work (chapters/themes) | Very good use of English used accurately in an academic style<br><br>Layout is attractive and reader friendly<br><br>The Harvard system is used consistently |
| 50–59 | Search strategy identified but lacks detailed justification<br><br>Less than comprehensive | The nature of the evidence included in the review is identified<br><br>Some of the studies included are critiqued showing good level of knowledge of research | Fairly clear links between concepts, theories and policy are demonstrated<br><br>Some implications for practice are identified | Area and focus to drive the review is fairly clear<br><br>Structure shows some links to the main focus | Good use of English used in a generally academic style<br><br>Layout is satisfactory |

| | | | | |
|---|---|---|---|---|
| | Some attempt to link strategy with main focus of review | | Logical progression would be improved by some restructuring | The Harvard system is used but with some inaccuracies/inconsistencies |
| 40–49 | Some elements of the search strategy unclear<br><br>Partial coverage of relevant literature in relation to the main focus of the review | Limited appreciation of the nature of the evidence included in the review<br><br>Some aspects of research understood and applied to critiquing some of the studies | Limited ability to demonstrate links between concepts, theories and policy<br><br>Limited attention to implications for practice | The area and focus not very clearly identified<br><br>Logical progression would be improved by some restructuring | Use of English is hindered by some syntax/typographical errors<br><br>Poor academic style<br><br>The Harvard system not adhered to well with many inaccuracies/inconsistencies |
| Below 39 | Search strategy not identified or unclear<br><br>Strategy not well justified<br><br>Identified literature inadequate to address the main focus of the review | Very limited evidence of critically examining the nature of the evidence utilized<br><br>Literature mainly described without critique | Disjointed presentation of ideas, not linked well together<br><br>Policy and practice relevance is not identified or developed | Unclear over main focus which should drive the review<br><br>Structure not coherent and not well justified<br><br>Disorganized presentation of the review | Very poor use of English seriously hinders clear communication of ideas<br><br>Poor adherence to the Harvard referencing system |

**Table 9.3** Breakdown of marks by category

| Category | Marks awarded in the range (%) |
| --- | --- |
| Searching the literature | 40–49 |
| Critical evaluation | 50–59 |
| Synthesis | below 40 |
| Organization and structure | 40–49 |
| Presentation | 60–69 |
| Total overall mark | 48 |

# Cue-consciousness

Developing a consciousness of the important elements within an assessment or any learning task will help you to effectively focus your efforts. In research by Miller and Parlett (1974:69) some students demonstrated a mature approach and were able to 'stand outside assessment situation, analyse it coolly and to decide how to cope with it'.

### Exercise 9.2

- Read Table 9.4 and identify which of the categories you resemble most
- In relation to a forthcoming assessment list all the cues you have from a range of sources
- Discuss and compare your list with a group of your peers
- Consider applications of the concept cue-sensitivity to learning and assessments other than exams
- Reflect on this exercise and devise a plan to improve your cue-consciousness if necessary

# Methods of assessment

In most courses which run for three years you will encounter a wide range of assessment methods often used in combination. Even in short courses and modules you may be assessed using some novel methods. Each should come with specific guidelines and unless there is explicit mention of choice and flexibility it

**Table 9.4** Cue-consciousness

| Category | Characteristics |
| --- | --- |
| Cue-conscious | Alertness to cues from lecturer concerning priorities for the end of year examinations |
| | Convinced that the impression the lecturer forms of the individual student is highly influential in their marking |
| | Believes there is a discernible technique in examinations |
| | Did well in examinations, often got upper second (2:1) in honours degree |
| | Reasonably confident in question-spotting, revises accordingly |
| | Success attributed to hard work and luck |
| Cue-seeker | As above but actively engaged in developing and exploiting relationships with lecturer |
| | Frequent social contact with lecturer probing for cues about their preferences and dislikes |
| | Important to be noticed through valuable contribution in classes and tutorials |
| | Narrowly focused revision strategy employed |
| | Believes that a high degree of control rests with the student |
| | Often got first class honours degree |
| | Confident in own abilities, any poor results attributed to poor technique |
| Cue-deaf | Believes the lecturer may form an impression of the individual student but this is incidental and insignificant |
| | If there is any technique or pattern to examinations it remains a mystery |
| | Not conscious of any cues about assessment |
| | Relies on hard work and wide coverage of the curriculum in revising for examinations |
| | Believes they have no control over the whole process of examinations |
| | Rigid view of 'right' and 'wrong' answers |
| | Generally received poor results in examinations and awarded significantly lower classification in their degree |
| | Failure is attributed to personal intellectual inadequacy |

is essential that you understand and adhere to exactly what is expected. Students have sometimes failed, not through lack of knowledge or ability, but because they did not understand what the set assessment required and relied on a third-hand interpretation from another student. The first prerequisites to success therefore are to:

- understand the expectations
- follow any specific guidelines provided by your lecturers.


# Planning for success in assessments

- Understand the remit – clarify your own interpretation and seek reassurance
- Timetable the work required – taking note of other priorities and the comparative weighting of the assessments
- Organize yourself – determine what information you need, where to obtain it and who you should work with – prepare your 'to do' list
- Keep a note of progress and resources as they are obtained and check relevance to the assessment task
- Take stock of your understanding of the topic. Have you got a grasp of the key points? Are you becoming clear on your position/arguments to put forward?
- Avoid trying to obtain all there is on a given topic – you will find that you have too many books and articles to cope with
- Stop collecting resources and start committing ideas to paper – write an overview plan of what the assignment will contain. Check this with any guidelines you have been provided with to ensure you remain on track
- Work on your first draft – use themes or sub-headings to clarify priorities and structure the piece of work. The format required for the eventual piece of work may not allow sub-headings but they will be invaluable at this stage
- Maintain a reference list as you use source material – leaving references till last has sometimes proved disastrous
- If tutorials or academic supervision is available do make use of it – it may not be possible to discover that your work is to the required standard before the marking process but it can be reassuring to know that your approach at least conforms to the general expectations
- If you have a safe study buddy or critical friend, deliver a draft to them for comment. You should wait until you have a draft that you are fairly satisfied with before doing this but ensure there is sufficient time to allow revisions before the submission deadline
- Revise your written work, check sufficient evidence and that your arguments are made logically, proofread for typographical errors, wrong words or spelling errors
- If you have detailed guidelines it will help if you can now tick each point to show you have attended to every detail

- After final polishing ensure you are using the prescribed format (e.g. style, font size, number of copies, word count), and complete the necessary paperwork. Submit using the required mode, e.g. online or bound hard copy, obtain proof and then forget it! Relax, you probably deserve it and no doubt need a rest!

While this generic advice applies to most methods of assessment it will be useful to have an overview of particular characteristics of different methods to help clarify specific expectations.

# Characteristics of assessment methods

### Essays and reports

These are pieces of writing which follow conventions. They are usually dictated by a set title presented supported by additional guidelines. Essays are covered in detail in Chapter 4 since this is a very common requirement in all nursing and midwifery courses. You should follow the conventions of academic writing. A report requires argumentation and support typical of an academic essay but the style and layout differ considerably. Headings or even numbering of main points will be expected.

### OSCE

This type of assessment, 'objective structured clinical examination', is used extensively in pre-registration courses and some CPD courses such as nurse prescribing. They may be held in clinical environments or 'training wards' but are often located in university clinical skills laboratories or interview rooms. A mock assessment is usually offered in preparation and, as with other methods, it would be very unwise not to make the most of this. Various scenarios will be set up in a circuit of assessment stations where you will be required to demonstrate a range of clinical practical skills to an examiner. The 'client' may be a real patient, a professional actor, or a staff or student volunteer. The examiner will often question your decision making and underlying knowledge supporting your competence but the time allocated for each student is short.

*Pointers for success*

- Comprehend the focus of the assessment
- Find out what the marking criteria are and obtain a copy of the marking grid in advance

- Rehearse the skills required and obtain reliable feedback in advance
- Relate these to situations where you have dealt with patients in practice
- Explore the evidence base
- Practise the OSCE
- Be prepared to self-assess after your performance at the OSCE

## Portfolio

The portfolio is very relevant to practice and according to Melrose (2006), represents an engaging method of assessment. You are likely to be required to submit a section of your portfolio, a profile, for assessment at various stages of your course. Pearce (2003) has shown that portfolios have been used in assessment to enable students to:

- provide evidence of achievement
- demonstrate professional competence
- achieve specified practice-based outcomes
- show critical reflection linking theory and practice.

The range of evidence will be made clear by your own institution but will typically include statements verified by mentors or clinical supervisors, learning contracts, testimonials, reflective accounts of practice and related learning, authoritative literature including research papers. These may be referred to as products of learning, items of evidence, artefacts or another related term.

### Pointers for success

- Requirements are sometimes complex, use tutorials to clarify exact requirements
- Ensure sufficient evidence is included but avoid making the document too bulky
- Professional appearance of the presentation is important, avoid cartoons and fancy fonts reminiscent of school projects
- Clearly organize and structure the portfolio – make it easy to use
- Use the terminology found in guidelines provided
- Links between theory and practice should be made explicit
- Highlight your achievements but do not neglect plans for future practice or additional learning needs you may have identified.

## Exams

These have traditionally been favoured since they demonstrate that what is produced is the student's own work but you will find that they are used very little in most nursing and midwifery courses. And while Rowntree (1977:135) points out that 'the 3-hour exam tests the students' ability to write at abnormal speeds, under unusual stress on someone else's topic without reference to his customary sources' you will still need to undertake exams and prepare well for them.

Examinations come in many formats including unseen, short answer, open book and multiple choice questions. The amount of information provided in advance varies and some allow materials: calculators, articles, dictionaries, into the exam room. Multiple choice questions (MCQ) may form part or all of the examination. Here you are presented with a short question along with four possible answers and you must select the correct one. This format is used for factual subjects like pharmacology.

### *Pointers for success*

- Check details regarding venue and times etc. and turn up with identification or other required documents
- Ensure you know the type of exam and its associated regulations well in advance and adhere to them
- Plan sufficient sleep in the days leading up to the exam
- Carefully devise a focused revision plan, collaborate with study buddies and attend any classes offered
- In view of Rowntree's (1977) observations, practise under precise conditions having obtained past papers – if the day of the exam is the first time you have had to write for three solid hours then you face an immediate disadvantage
- For MCQs there are numerous books and Internet sites providing examples giving invaluable practise with almost instant feedback

## Video analysis

Here you may be given a short section of video and instructed to write an analysis. This may be a scenario where bad news is conveyed, a counselling interview, or history taking in a family planning clinic. You will then need to use relevant theoretical frameworks or research evidence to support your judgements on the merit of aspects of the video scenario. This is then submitted in the form of a report.

### *Pointers for success*

- View the video several times and consider using the SQ3R technique
- Much of the generic advice applies
- Ensure the framework or research you use is appropriate and be explicit in linking this to the video clip

*Poster presentation*

A poster is simply a static, visual medium (usually of the paper and board variety) that you use to communicate ideas and messages. It will relate to a topic directed to some extent by your lecturers. A display of work may be organized as part of an end of year conference and peer assessment may be utilized. Often a written justification will be required in addition to the poster itself.

- Seek help from within the university, e.g. a resources unit may offer material help and advice
- Ensure you are aware of which aspects form part of the assessment, it may be the quality of the display or just the written report
- Consult published guides for advice on layout etc. (Jackson and Sheldon, 2000)

## Viva or oral examination

This adds variety to assessment and authenticates students' work. It may allow compensation in a given part of the course and the effort and attainment during the viva may make the difference between a pass and fail. Some courses will allow for students to be asked to attend a viva where there are queries about an assignment. Many expect all students to be assessed in this way. You may be asked to defend a dissertation, case study or entries in a profile submitted previously.

*Pointers for success*

- Practise any presentation you must give
- Devise obscure and obvious questions which may be asked in relation to the work you have produced. Ensure you have research-based answers ready
- Be utterly familiar with work previously submitted
- Take water with you

## Dissertation

This is likely to be the biggest piece of work you may need to submit and it could be the component which gives your course its honours status. However, the term 'dissertation' covers a very broad range of assignments, of possibly between 5,000 and 80,000 words. In first degree programmes the maximum word limit is likely to be 10,000 words where a double module is undertaken for the dissertation. If this is the assessment method for your PhD, it will fall at the upper end of this scale and you are advised to consult specific texts offering tailored advice (Phillips and Pugh, 2005). Most dissertations are simply part of your degree course requiring an in-depth extended essay, research proposal or literature review – academic assignments which attract specific supervision arrangements that are largely covered elsewhere in this book.

### Pointers for success

- Make use of the supervision available
- Keep accurate records of decisions and advice from supervision sessions
- Time management is vital; plan backwards from the submission date and set key targets

# Plagiarism

It is good to see students doing well in assessments. I remember an examination board where one student midwife had been given around 80% for some coursework. The lecturers were delighted but just before the mark was agreed the external examiner spoke. She was delighted too that the work had been given a high mark, but questioned if the student deserved the grade. She produced an article from her bag and proceeded to show about 50% of the student's essay was copied directly from it. It had in fact been published by this external examiner! This student was qualified and there was discussion about informing her manager and the NMC since plagiarism amounts to fraud. If somebody is prepared to cheat in the university setting perhaps they will falsify clinical records or display other aspects of dishonesty in their professional practice!

All universities say that plagiarism is a serious matter and for many it carries penalties which demonstrate its seriousness. Estimates concerning the prevalence of plagiarism vary but it is agreed that the problem is considerable and of particular concern in courses associated with nursing or midwifery, which carries professional obligations to uphold public trust.

Several measures have been put in place to avoid, deter or detect plagiarism, such as:

- explicit teaching on this topic and clear policies reiterated in course materials
- signature required with a declaration that submissions are the student's own work
- requirement to submit work online or in electronic format to allow the use of plagiarism detection software
- clear advice regarding learning activities in groups, i.e. never to share files with colleagues.

## Difficult circumstances

It is well recognized that life events and stresses may interfere with your ability to learn and hinder your performance in assessments. Many students cope with very difficult circumstances and through hard work, support from friends and others, engaging with the university and adopting efficient learning strategies, they succeed almost against all the odds. Each department will have policies which assist in genuine difficulties. These must usually relate to circumstances which are unexpected, beyond your control and have a detrimental impact on your ability to study at a time crucial for assessments or related learning. Do read your university polices which will explain the sort of things that may be considered.

University staff and university policy will generally be supportive of students who experience genuine difficulties. Behind the scenes however there is a raft of forms and administrative procedures and so it is wise to keep in touch with the lecturers concerned. Where you could anticipate a problem go and talk this over well in advance as this will enable paperwork to be prepared in advance.

Often the decision concerning a request for special consideration is a joint one involving a panel of academic staff.

Your request must be made:

- using the appropriate form (may be online)
- within the prescribed time frame, usually before a submission date
- and accompanied by sufficient evidence.

Examples of reasons offered for special consideration:

- Horse had colic
- Had to buy a new car and moved house
- Could not open data stick
- 'I panicked, realized I had not revised and ran out of the exam room'
- Was arrested for being drunk
- Grandmother was admitted to ITU and died
- Laptop was stolen

Some may evoke understanding while others may evoke the disciplinary procedure! Even where there is bereavement it may prove ineligible unless it was at a crucial period. The problem with the horse was accepted but it has been known for a student to have around eight grandmothers die during a three-year period! While it may prove impossible you should try to obtain some form of evidence to support your claims. Contact with your personal tutor or academic supervisor may be a source of support and they may then be able to corroborate your claim and support your request at the appropriate panel or examination board. Often students who do have sufficient reason and are granted an extension actually go on to submit on time or do not use their full extension period. It may be worth applying as a safeguard when difficulties occur.

The outcome of your request may be:

- Denial – Here the evidence may be unconvincing or outside the policy guidelines and is thus rejected, any penalties you hoped to avoid will be applied.
- Extension – You may be granted a new submission date, providing an additional week or more for coursework or given an additional attempt at an examination.
- Deferral – A very lengthy extension where your coursework may be required at the same time as the cohort behind you, e.g. 6 months. You may have to change groups and complete your course later than expected.
- Mitigating circumstances – May be considered at an examination board and allow the attempt to be discounted or considered void. This will mean that your second submission will be counted as your first attempt.

# Springboard to success

Some students who get 65% view this as failure. They did not live up to their expectations, or possibly the expectations of others! A result below the pass standard or your own expectations can be helpful since you will be forced to analyse what went wrong.

If you feel strongly that your work deserved more credit since you spent virtually all night revising and are certain that you deserved to pass, there are a few options open to you:

1 Appeal via the established system which is usually time limited and only open where approved 'grounds for appeal' exist
2 Write to the Vice Chancellor, your MP and the local newspaper about the injustice
3 Arrive unannounced at the office of the person who marked the work to have it out with them
4 Carefully read the feedback provided, often a word-processed compilation complemented by written comments on your paper which is returned to you
5 Revisit the assessment guide and analyse your efforts and achievement in the light of these

6  Attend any revision classes or tutorials on offer
7  Book into specific student support groups, e.g. academic writing support, details of which can be obtained via student services.

Option 1 is rarely called for but this is your right and the university must make the process clear. Option 2 may get you noticed but in 20 years experience I cannot recall a single case when this was justified! Option 3 will undoubtedly be unproductive especially if you arrive in an angry state. Options 4, 5, 6 and 7 are likely to be useful and may also put you in touch with support systems. There is usually a requirement to provide specific feedback, which should serve at least two key purposes. It should justify the grade awarded in relation to known criteria and it should indicate how the work could be developed and improved. If the feedback is illegible or difficult to decipher and appears not to fulfil these key functions you may then approach the lecturer for an appointment to receive clarification.

Comparing your results with peers and engaging in a morbid post-mortem may lead to efforts to correct what you see as an injustice, convinced that your work was marked by a 'hard marker'. While occasionally things do go wrong and assessments are rendered unfair, in general the sense of injustice and the fraught tutorials where your goal is to change the grade, are ineffectual. What may be more productive is to use the experience as a springboard to success in the second attempt and transfer the insights and skills developed to ensure first time successes in future assessments.

## Conclusion

This chapter has provided numerous pointers for success in assessments that you face on your nursing or midwifery course. Key amongst these is the need to fully grasp what the requirements are; developing sensitivity to the available cues will assist in this process. You can then engage in meaningful preparation. Most students pass most things at the first attempt but occasionally this is not the case. The feedback you obtain will then be vital to use this experience as a springboard to future success. Assessment is also about learning and should not be viewed as a separate activity. Your preparation will result in learning and the feedback, even where you do very well, will confirm your learning and can also highlight how to obtain even better results in future.

# Part 5

Expertise for success:
the lifelong learner in
nursing and midwifery

# 10

# Career pathways in nursing and midwifery

*Introduction • Transition • Orientation programmes • Career mentor*
*• New roles and opportunities in professional practice • Keeping informed*
*• Conclusions*

This chapter is very different from the others and is quite unusual in that it is short. Much of the content however has been lodged on a free website and many of the topics covered deserve serious consideration by readers who are embarking on their professional career, changing direction or mapping out their career pathway. Similarly, all of the exercises, which help you to see the relevance of these topics for yourself, are on the website.

👉 www.openup.co.uk/nursing success. You will see this icon again to prompt you that there is more web material on a given area.

Here the important transition from 'student' to 'qualified' is given consideration and advice on how to keep this in perspective and cope well. Orientation programmes offered to new employees will be instrumental in making this process exciting and enjoyable and offer a lifeline to those who feel they are thrown into the deep end. In the medium- to long-term in your career the career mentor will be useful and CPD students may skip straight to this section. New roles and opportunities, increasing in both nursing and midwifery, are also covered.

On the website there is material to support you in devising your personal development plan and much detail on how to secure the post you want, including:

- curriculum vitae
- covering letter
- job description
- person specification
- application form
- job interview.

# Introduction

You may be approaching the end of your course. The relief of its completion is in sight. If you are already qualified, though the transition may not be as great as for your newly qualified colleagues in nursing or midwifery, there is still much to be gained from this chapter. At the completion of a recent community specialist practice course, a full-time 12-month course, several students were set on quite unexpected career pathways. Some who had been seconded had no posts to return to, others were taking up new initiatives requiring additional language skills which they happened to have and one secured employment teaching child development in further education. There are many varied opportunities for full- or part-time careers within all branches of nursing and midwifery. Some take pathways initially out of necessity or, apparently, by chance. However, being prepared, having goals and working towards them will enable you to be in a position to steer your own career pathway, to make opportunities or be ready to take opportunities as they present themselves. Part of that preparation includes devising your personal development plan, maintaining your CV and seeking new opportunities. Here you should visit the website for advice.

# Transition

Following hard on the heels of your success on recent courses comes the excitement of a first or a new post in nursing or midwifery. For the newly qualified this first year presents a steep learning curve. You may be adequately prepared for the academic award and looking forward to renewing acquaintances at your awards ceremony. You may be adequately prepared to enter the register held by the Nursing and Midwifery Council and eagerly awaiting official notification after parting with your first year's registration fee. The first year also holds in store a time of change; a chance to consolidate your learning; but many newly qualified nurses and midwives feel quite unprepared when faced with their new responsibilities. You will however develop confidence in your own decision making, form relationships, establish networks and perhaps develop your career plan.

It is a time of transition which, when measured on a stress scoring system used extensively in research by Cohen *et al.* (1997), is not insignificant. In addition to the normal stressors one could expect in an average year there are those which accompany this first year in a professional role, and even if you are expert in supporting clients, perhaps as a qualified psychiatric nurse, I am afraid this does not confer immunity.

Life events, which may accompany your success on midwifery or nursing courses, include:

- Some valued relationships, established over 3 or more years, will inevitably alter or even end
- Moving to new accommodation, perhaps relocating
- New financial commitments and responsibilities
- Becoming familiar with a new professional role
- Accountability for your own professional practice
- Having to adjust to a new team of colleagues and establish your credibility
- The demand to fully participate in a rotation system, which may include a lengthy block of nights.

Do bear in mind that, particularly on pre-registration courses, you have survived many changes in getting to your current position, and although this is markedly different, you have already proved you can do it. A positive approach and a willingness to seek advice and use the networks of support, both formal and informal, make this time of transition a valuable experience where you are able to develop in confidence based on evidence. The evidence of feedback from patients, colleagues and supervisors which confirms your professional competence is based on your underpinning knowledge base.

Many features built into your employment contract and conditions of service facilitate the transition to qualified nurse or midwife. Make sure you engage with these, as they will serve to introduce you to key policies, practices and key people within your new organization.

# Orientation programmes

These differ between organizations; often there will be a generic element supplemented by a more specific element. The orientation programme will take you away from your new place of employment, perhaps to the plush administration building of your organization. Here you will enjoy keeping office hours, free corporate sandwiches and a mass of new information. Key however will be the opportunity to meet people from different departments who will be drafted in to lead some of the presentations and many new recruits from diverse occupations such as porters and security, nuclear medicine, physiotherapy and even volunteers. This little group, meeting together for just a few days, may well initially form an important informal support network. Over the months you can ring them with your naïve questions without embarrassment. Just a friendly greeting, exchanged on chance meetings along the miles of corridor, may be reassuring.

The specific element of your orientation may involve further meetings with key people and even a prescribed set of competencies to be worked through with a designated supervisor. While you may feel this process to be unnecessary, it is a safeguard to the organization and provides valuable revision or new learning for you which can be reassuring. The orientation is for your benefit, ultimately to enable you to make an effective contribution to enhancing patient care and achieving the corporate goals of your employer. Therefore it is reasonable for you to direct the process to some extent and make specific requests to include additional features to the orientation programme. The needs will be specific to both you and the post but the following provides illustrations from various disciplines:

- Commencing as a staff nurse in an orthopaedic ward, a half day placement in the plaster department may prove very valuable
- Taking up a new midwifery post, it is reasonable for the post holder to develop a working acquaintance with the gynaecology department
- Working in a hospital-at-home team for sick children will mean familiarization with the child protection team
- Being employed as a learning disabilities nurse in a community-based charity offering employment to clients will require a working relationship with all referring agencies.

Keeping a reflective diary, by now second nature to many, is not something to be disposed of as you collect your diploma or receive your NMC PIN number. It will be invaluable during this period but perhaps of more immediate importance is the need for a blank notebook to record vital information and key questions. This was essential equipment for John Fowler when newly qualified (Fowler, 2005). He recently led a team of practice educators in writing a useful book containing 5-minute answers to over 70 frequently asked questions. While there is some emphasis on adult nursing there are many entries of importance to newly qualified staff across all nursing and midwifery boundaries.

# Career mentor

Towards the end of the pre-registration course you will be utterly familiar with the concept of mentor. CPD students may also have benefited from good mentors but are more probably familiar with taking that role themselves. Your mentors may have measured up well to the idealized characteristics:

- wise and kindly experienced midwife or nurse
- trusted adviser
- educator and guide
- nurturing and role modelling
- personal integrity.

The reality however may have been more varied and your mentor is likely to have been enlisted for a short term focused on achievement of specific competencies. There are nevertheless many excellent nurses and midwives who have done exceptionally well in their careers and who may offer examples and role models for those following similar career pathways.

Career mentoring holds 'great potential for enhancing career success' (Baugh and Sullivan, 2005: 425) which has been shown to help protégés by increasing:

- job satisfaction and career mobility
- awareness of developmental opportunities
- individuals' ability to meet some of the challenges to advancement (Baugh and Sullivan, 2005: 502).

McAlearney (2005: 500), who surveyed chief executives found around three-quarters had 'sought developmental relationships with informal mentors both within and outside their organizations' while less than a quarter had any formal mentoring. So while there is unlikely to be a formal career mentoring system, especially at the beginning of your career, it is worth seeking such a beneficial relationship.

# New roles and opportunities in professional practice

While most nurses or midwives soon begin to appreciate the very wide scope for developing their careers, and even during their pre-registration training period meet an array of specialists and non-traditional practitioners, the image of nursing in the public mind remains archaic.

The context of health care and the need for nursing and midwifery services is constantly developing, influenced by numerous factors, and each of these will shape the career development opportunities you will face. They are too numerous to mention but include:

- greater community focus and long-term conditions
- disease prevention and the development of public health
- e-health and remote monitoring of patients
- high priority on keeping people out of hospital, e.g. 'hospital at home'
- independent midwifery practice
- patient and public expectations, partnership, choice and involvement.

The Department of Health (2006b:3) recognizes that 'some will choose to climb an upward ladder of increasing responsibility and higher reward, many other nurses choose a more lateral career journey, moving within and between care groups and settings' and this applies equally to midwives. The recent introduction of community matrons to provide an opportunity for experienced nurses to advance their skills so that they can make a difference to the lives of patients with long-term conditions, is one example of keeping highly skilled nurses close to patient care.

New forms of practitioner have recently emerged such as emergency care practitioners (ECP) and surgeons' assistants, which may attract nurses. The experienced paediatric nurse who makes a lateral move to become an ECP may then find that upward progression is rapid and without challenge. Likewise some of the developing professions such as operating department practitioners (ODP) may provide unique opportunities for nurses or midwives who possess joint qualifications.

# Keeping informed

There are frequently published nursing and midwifery journals that advertise new posts and courses, with more senior posts also appearing in quality daily newspapers. A useful booklet, *TARGET Nursing & Midwifery*, published annually by GTI Specialist Publishers not only provides a guide for newly qualified nurses and midwives but includes many career profiles. This publication, obtainable free from your local careers service or university library is supplemented by a regularly updated website (doctorjob.com/nursing) packed with advice.

**Other useful mechanisms to keep informed include:**

- networking and keeping in touch with former fellow students now dispersed
- jobs fairs, organized regularly by the Royal College of Midwifery and the Royal College of Nursing
- NHS daily e-mail notification system to suit the parameters you select
- conferences, especially large events, with numerous employers in attendance
- armed forces and overseas organizations
- private sector employees and charities which employ professional qualified staff.

# Conclusions

If you have not yet started to plan your career then the time to start is now. Preparation is vital and if you are goal-directed you are more likely to achieve your aspirations than if you drift along with the tides. There are numerous sources of guidance; key among these will be your career mentor so be alert for such a person. Others such as websites and conferences will help you keep informed of opportunities, but expect to take charge yourself, seek opportunities and make these happen.

The website linked to this chapter provides additional links to help you keep informed. Whether you develop laterally or upward ensure you do not stand still, for the sake of your clients if not yourself.

# 11

# Lifelong learning organizations and CPD to sustain your professional practice

*Introduction • Lifelong learning in context • Concepts examined*
*• Professional requirements • Demonstrating PREP (CPD) standards*
*• Framework for lifelong learning • Informal/unstructured learning activities*
*• Protected time • Support from professional organizations • In-person*
*support • Midwives and supervision • Special interests and opportunities*
*• Formal structured learning • Using information technology to facilitate LLL*
*• RSS News Feeds • Blogs • Discussion lists • Conclusions*

This chapter examines the important concepts 'lifelong learning' (LLL) and CPD and what they mean for nurses and midwives. The professional obligation on individuals to become lifelong learners is outlined along with an explanation of how to demonstrate achievement of post-registration education and practice (PREP) standards. A framework for lifelong learning is examined and later returned to and used in extended exercises focusing on factors which contribute to your own LLL. Numerous exciting opportunities to engage in CPD, most of which do not involve attending formal courses of study, are explored. 'Protected time' for nurses and midwives to engage in professional development is examined and encouraged. Various mechanisms of support are explored and midwifery supervision is examined as a key motivator in LLL. Development of a special interest is illustrated with a case study from the area of multiple sclerosis nursing. Both formal and informal learning opportunities are covered along with the contribution of information technology to professional CPD.

## Introduction

Lifelong learning is something which will enhance your enjoyment and make your career more satisfying and rewarding. It is something which all nursing and midwifery organizations, NHS Trusts, Primary Care Trusts, independent health care providers and governing bodies are committed to. The fact that you are on a course, a secondment or enjoying some measure of support may be evidence of your organization's commitment to lifelong learning along with your own commitment to professional standards. Whilst there is an understandable relief on completion of a period of study, and some midwifery and nursing students are uploading their textbooks onto an Internet auction site to mark the end of their studying, the reality is that initial qualification marks a period of intense learning. Jarvis (2005:658) argued that study skills should be an integral part of professional courses, in part to make the whole process efficient, but also to enable professionals to become 'effective lifelong learners'.

The Department of Health (2004b:8) recommends that learning should be viewed as a 'continuum from pre- to post-qualifying education and CPD'. Likewise, taking on a new or enhanced professional role requires ongoing learning. If you have worked through most of the chapters of this book, engaged in many of the exercises and developed efficient study habits you are well equipped with many of the tools for lifelong learning and CPD.

## Lifelong learning in context

Whether your career involves 'moving within and between care groups and settings' (Department of Health, 2006b: 3), branching into research or education, or moving in a linear route up the management ladder, you will need to engage in

LLL activities. Even in the following examples the need for learning and development remains:

- part-time midwife who remains attached to a community health centre for several decades
- nurse doing just one night per week in an old age psychiatric ward.

In the extreme a nurses or midwives who neglect this obligation put their registration at risk and may face legal consequences if their patients are put at risk. However, many nurses and midwives maintain a spirit of enquiry and keen interest in their professions which naturally leads to embracing a lifelong learning ethos and the enjoyment of ongoing curiosity-led learning.

The NHS aims to foster a learning culture and is committed to the view that 'investment in learning benefits the organization, patients and carers, local communities, society more generally and individuals' (Department of Health, 2001:6). This is strengthened by making explicit links between education and development, and career and pay progression through the Knowledge and Skills Framework (KSF) and Agenda for Change (Department of Health, 2004c).


## Concepts examined

Lifelong learning and CPD are concepts that have been used interchangeably. However, Wilcox (2005) has made a distinction between them by suggesting that LLL is the all-embracing umbrella term whereas CPD is but one of its spokes. CPD is seen as 'the means to keep you up-to-date, safe and competent as a practitioner' (Wilcox, 2005:44), with the possibility of individual benefits such as maintaining your:

- interest and satisfaction,
- employability,
- career prospects.

The Department of Health (1998) defined lifelong learning as 'a process of continuing development for all individuals and teams which meets the needs of patients and delivers the health care outcomes and health care priorities of the NHS, and which enables professionals to expand and fulfil their potential'.

It later made the focus of lifelong learning clear in stating that it 'is primarily about growth and opportunity, about making sure staff are supported to acquire new skills and realize their potential to help change things for the better'

(Department of Health, 2001:1). By way of practical support it suggests that 'continuing professional development must be part of the process of lifelong learning for all health care professionals – its purpose is to help professionals care for patients ... it must be supported by the NHS and by the professions' (Department of Health, 2001:37). Numerous policy level statements offer support for CPD and LLL in health care but it is worth noting that supporting the individual development of nurses and midwives is instrumental in delivering core objectives of the NHS (Department of Health, 2004a).

## Exercise 11.1

- Identify as many reasons for engaging in CPD as you can
- Consider the pressures you feel to become a lifelong learner and where these emerge from
- Who may benefit from nurses and midwives becoming lifelong learners?

As a midwife or nurse you are obliged by virtue of your employment contract to attend mandatory annual updates. You may have identified this from the exercise above along with numerous pressures or reasons for going well beyond this mandatory minimum. Compare your list with the one below, offered as possible driving forces promoting lifelong learning in nursing and midwifery.

- Changes in
  - health care needs of the population
  - professional roles
  - therapeutic approaches/technologies
- Individual
  - career enhancement/promotion
  - responsibilities
  - knowledge or skills deficits
  - impact of evidence-based nursing and midwifery practice
- Professional
  - mentoring future students (perhaps including those from other disciplines)
  - role developments and expansion
- Public concerns over
  - quality of care
  - safety for patients/clients

Notice how many of these factors listed relate to change of one type or another. Learning, you will recall, is a change in behaviour, attitudes or knowledge that is relatively permanent and is essential for successfully managing change. This is one of the key official motivators in supporting lifelong learning within the NHS;

it is seen as vitally instrumental in delivering policy agendas using its staff as the main resource. 'Post qualifying learning' and CPD are seen as 'critical for the delivery of:

- The NHS Plan
- National Service Frameworks
- Clinical governance (Department of Health, 2004a:3).

It is worth bearing this emphasis in mind when planning for your own LLL to ensure there is support from policy level statements, at least to some extent.


# Professional requirements

The Nursing and Midwifery Council, as part of its overall remit to protect the public, require all registrants to renew their registration every three years. In order to do so they must comply with the PREP (practice) standards and the PREP (CPD) standards. PREP is a self-verification system but registrants must be prepared to submit relevant evidence to the NMC if this is requested.

The current (2007) practice standard requires nurses, midwives and specialist community public health nurses (health visitors) renewing their registration to confirm that they have undertaken at least 450 hours of practice over the preceding three years for each registration they wish to renew. The current CPD standard requires nurses, midwives and specialist community public health nurses to confirm that they have undertaken 35 hours of relevant learning activity during the preceding three years. They are also required to record this learning; there is a suggested format for this (Nursing and Midwifery Council, 2006a:10). Many people have more than one recorded qualification, for instance a specialist community public health nurse may maintain a part-time or bank post in mental health nursing and would therefore need to maintain these standards in each field.

This scheme provides assurances to the public that all registrants have maintained at least the minimum standard. If registration lapses you will not be able to be employed legally as a nurse or midwife. These standards change from time to time so it is important that you read the regular NMC newsletter which is sent to all registrants, read *The PREP Handbook* (Nursing and Midwifery Council, 2006b) and seek advice from the NMC if you have specific queries (http://www.nmc-uk.org/). After any lengthy break from practice it is again vital to check these standards as you may be required to undertake an approved 'return to practice' course in order for your registration to become reactivated.

# Demonstrating PREP (CPD) standards

The Nursing and Midwifery Council (2006a:3) describes the best thing about PREP as: 'it is entirely up to you how to meet the standards', providing a great deal of flexibility and scope to individual practitioners. It is worth reiterating that there is no such thing as an approved learning activity and most nurses and midwives achieve the standards by engaging in informal learning activities. Guiding principles dictate that it must be relevant to your work, or the work you intend to do in the near future and it must assist you to provide the highest possible standards of care to your clients or patients.

*The PREP Handbook* has 17 detailed examples of learning activities drawn from a range of fields of nursing practice and midwifery; they are almost equally divided between structured/formal and unstructured/informal activities. In line with reflection on practice, the important thing to remember in undertaking CPD activities for the purpose of PREP is that you must be able to articulate both the outcome of your learning and how the learning relates to your work.

### Exercise 11.2

- Think about three learning activities you have engaged in over the past 12 months
- Remember these do not have to be formal study days etc. and may relate to incidents from your personal life
- Consider for each of these what learning has taken place and how this relates to your work
- Select one of the activities and discuss it with a colleague (preceptor, supervisor, study buddy)
- Could you record the number of hours the activity took and use this as part of your evidence of achieving the CPD standards?

# Framework for lifelong learning

Gopee (2005) has developed a framework for lifelong learning from his PhD studies, which places the practitioner at the centre but crucially involves three important factors related to:

- the socio-political climate

- organizations
- personal or individual issues.

All of these contribute to the need for lifelong learning in nursing and midwifery and may serve to encourage practitioners to respond positively to the demands.

At times, for instance when there are atypical financial constraints, the climate may prove less favourable to those wishing to fully engage in lifelong learning. While it is possible to fulfil the minimum professional requirements without significant monetary cost, there may be other hidden costs and inevitably all nurses and midwives will require some developments which do involve fee payment. For some years, nurses and midwives have been undertaking CPD in their own time, which threatens a healthy work–life balance and recently there are concerns that CPD funding may be diverted.

Some organizations are always sending their staff on study days. The organizational climate at management, unit or small team level will each exert its distinctive influence, and even within the same organization these may be quite different. At an official level there will be clear endorsement of the aims and aspirations of LLL. This may or may not be complemented by a real commitment and enthusiasm amongst senior managers, training and research staff and senior midwives and nurses. However, it does not naturally follow that the same positive views will be equally evident at the unit, ward or team level. You will recall a variety of learning environments which formed part of the circuit of clinically-based placements; similar variations should be anticipated. In some teams constraints may be so tangible that your first decision may be to devise an exit strategy and be much more careful in investigating the ethos of your next post before accepting it! Many areas are however genuinely supportive of LLL and CPD activities, offering as much practical and financial support as possible.

Individual nurses and midwives will have many life roles which change across the lifespan and with shifting personal circumstances. These will inevitably impact on their commitment, ability and extent to which they can engage in LLL activities. Being full-time professional and part-time carer leaves limited capacity or energy for anything above the minimum. While all registrants are obliged to meet the PREP (CPD) standard, many will undertake more than the minimum making it necessary to be selective when considering your NMC documentation.

# Informal/unstructured learning activities

There are numerous activities within one's own sphere of responsibility, which occur during working hours, to provide real learning and development opportunities. These include:

- taking on roles and responsibilities, e.g.:
  - liaison role with others within and beyond the traditional multidisciplinary team
  - ordering equipment and evaluating new products
  - presenting a poster with others, at a Trust-wide conference
  - cascade trainer, e.g. in breakaway techniques or infection control
- undertaking:
  - an audit of practice
  - a demonstration or short teaching session
  - guiding a newly appointed healthcare assistant
  - looking up information on a new or unfamiliar drug and disseminating details to colleagues
  - supervision of students
- active involvement with:
  - a research project
  - a special interest or project group
  - setting up a new service or therapy
  - a journal club where you read, reflect and report on an article or editorial
  - observing episodes of clinical care and discussing these with colleagues.

In addition numerous informal events which occur outside your workplace will also potentially result in valuable learning. Consider the list below:

- attending a place of worship where British Sign Language interpretation is provided
- conversations with a speaker at a conference
- dealing with the funeral arrangements for a family member
- engaging with IT directed by teenage son or daughter
- joining a local gym
- learning about ethnic cookery from a friend
- visiting an elderly relative in an acute hospital setting
- visiting other departments or centres of excellence
- watching a documentary on TV
- writing for the 'opinion column' or letters page of a newspaper or professional journal.

Clearly all of these may result in learning but at first glance the relevance to nursing or midwifery may be less apparent. However, depending on the field of practice, each one could have relevance and you may be able to give an account of how the learning relates to your work. If so it is quite probable that, with a little imagination, all of these activities could be used to fulfil part of the PREP (CPD) standards.

# Protected time

There are well-known barriers to LLL:

- time or sufficient paid leave for learning of various kinds
- financial support for courses/study days etc.
- adequate cover in clinical practice to release staff or for staff to feel comfortable leaving colleagues or clients.

A statutory duty for allied health professionals to undertake CPD was introduced in 2006 and this adds to the growing demand by nurses and midwives for 'protected time' (White, 2006). For some years occupational therapists have been given a minimum half-day per month for development related work. A recent study found that 'undertaking regular CPD within the workplace improved staff morale and recruitment and retention' (White, 2006:440). These factors and a growing recognition of the need for CPD are beginning to result in increasing the provision of protected time. This may form part of the contract of employment of senior or specialist midwives and nurses but in some areas protected time is becoming the norm for all staff. While it may be used effectively to engage in some of the work-based or informal activities listed above, the case study described below shows an approach where the focus is specific to local needs and requires attendance at a series of work-based sessions.

### The Protected Learning Time Programme: an example.

The Welsh Rural Postgraduate Unit and Local Health Board Powys (N.D.) introduced this programme in 2005. One of the aims was to ensure a rapid response to new technological and governance issues within health care and the NHS which supports its focus on local delivery of services.

The programme will:

- provide one afternoon per month of protected learning time for all professionals and staff working in general practice/primary care in Powys

- cover the whole of Powys
- form part of an annual rolling programme of CPD in Powys for primary care
- provide cover for all participating practices for the duration of the afternoon sessions (1pm–6pm)
- cater for the needs of doctors, nurses (practice nurses and other attached nursing staff), allied health professionals, and administration and managerial staff.

## Exercise 11.3

According to the conceptual framework for lifelong learning proposed by Gopee (2005), insufficient input from any of the three key factors may diminish the effectiveness and implementation of lifelong learning. This exercise is in three parts and focuses on socio-political, organizational and individual factors.

### Socio-political factors

Investigate the current socio-political environment in which nursing and midwifery occurs.

- Obtain and read recent Department of Health policy documents and initiatives, available via the extensive Department of Health website http://www.dh.gov.uk/home/fs/en
- Consider present government policies related to the economy, education and health and their impact on nursing and midwifery
- Scan recent NHS related news (professional journals and BBC News online health section and archives will facilitate this) http://news.bbc.co.uk/
- Having completed the above identify and reflect on the factors influencing lifelong learning and answer the following questions: Is the climate generally supportive or hostile? Which policies or initiatives can you currently use to support your CPD needs?

### Organizational factors

Investigate your own organization's stance on lifelong learning and CPD.

- Discuss informally with colleagues and at team meetings
- Obtain and read the corporate business plan and any departmental plans which complement this – read this questioningly focusing on learning and CPD issues
- Identify the policy on 'protected time' for health professionals and compare professional disciplines
- Take note of local and regional press reports about NHS provisions and

plans which will include both reshaping or reductions in services and the development of new services
- Reflect on the factors which emerge and consider the extent to which your own CPD plans coincide with local goals and initiatives

### Individual factors

You will inevitably find that you are engaged in some form of CPD activity each year in your role as a midwife or nurse.

- Identify the opportunities and mandatory events provided by your employer; get a copy of their flyer or consult their web pages
- Reflect on your current role and areas of development you need in order to attain and maintain competencies
- Are your needs met by the routine CPD provisions made by your current employer?
- Reflect on both the socio-political and organizational factors and how these impact on your needs and aspirations and discuss this with your 'career mentor'
- Devise a tentative short-term action plan and discuss this with key individuals such as your line manager or midwifery or clinical supervisor

## Support from professional organizations

The Royal College of Nursing (RCN), with around 390,000 members in 2007, holds a major annual congress spanning the best part of a week which provides lively debate, networking opportunities and numerous educational events. It also offers over 100 forums covering all nursing disciplines and also has a Midwifery Society. Members can join these groups and will receive regular newsletters and access to specific online materials. Non-members can attend forum events which include an annual conference bringing together a network of colleagues with similar interests and CPD needs, national leaders, researchers and experts within their fields.

The range and degree of specialization is remarkable as this small sample of forum titles illustrates:

- children and young people mental health
- health visitors and public health
- in-flight nurses
- learning disability nursing
- mental health practice

- neurosciences
- nursing students
- paediatric oncology
- pain forum.

Many of these forums have developed specific competency frameworks (Parkinson's Disease Society, 2005) which can be used to identify and direct development needs. Some are supported by a related professional journal; these usually carry specific interactive articles designed to promote learning and which are designated for the purpose of CPD. The *Nursing Standard*, an RCN weekly journal, carries one such article in every issue.

Consultant nurse networks are also facilitated. In addition the RCN has numerous regional resource centres offering library facilities, Internet access, journal collections and other learning resources, some of which are open to non-members. (www.rcn.org.uk)

# In-person support

Within the NHS nurses and midwives are expected to have an annual development review meeting with their manager. Managers are key in facilitating staff development so it is important that you prepare for this review (Royal College of Nursing, 2006).

Preceptorship is becoming more widespread and organizations are using it as an incentive for prospective employees. Following the implementation of Agenda for Change this has gathered impetus. For some staff groups such as nursing and occupational therapy, band 5 is the entry point for newly qualified staff and preceptorship is part of a professional framework to ease the transition from the role of student to the role of qualified practitioner.

The overall aims of preceptorship are to:

- provide valuable support during the early phase of taking up a band 5 post
- facilitate the development of knowledge, skills and professional behaviour
- assist new band 5 entrants to identify evidence to support the achievement of their foundation KSF outline and to work with their supervisor to identify an appropriate personal development plan.

Beyond the transition period ongoing clinical supervision should be offered to all nurses as a formal process of professional support aimed at enabling practitioners to:

- develop their knowledge and competence
- assume responsibility for their own practice
- enhance client safety in complex situations.

There are many models of clinical supervision in operation and you need to invest in the relationship with your supervisor to make this work for you (Nursing and Midwifery Council, 2006c). Your supervisor will be a more experienced nurse and can provide invaluable advice in particular circumstances and help with your CPD needs and aspirations, linked explicitly to your place of employment.


## Midwives and supervision

Many of the issues and key factors supporting LLL apply equally to nurses and midwives but some CPD provision must be discipline-specific. A recent abstract (Day-Stirk, 2006:372) highlighted the need for midwives to exercise assertiveness in relation to their accountability which stems from midwives' well-established professional autonomy. These issues are by no means new but since they remain live this reinforces the need for midwives to embrace the ethos of lifelong learning.

Around 95% of practising midwives join the Royal College of Midwives (RCM), which runs an active CPD programme. It offers study days, lectures, interactive clinical workshops, courses, conferences and open learning materials as well as providing accreditation for educational events provided by other organizations. The thrust of this programme is to help midwives meet their mandatory PREP requirements and to enhance skills supporting the goal of maintaining and improving standards of care for mothers and babies (Royal College of Midwives, 2006).

Midwifery has a long-established system of self-regulation that directly impacts on each individual midwife as enshrined in the *Midwives Rules and Standards* (Nursing and Midwifery Council, 2004b). The statutory supervision of midwives is a UK-wide requirement. It places each midwife in a relationship with a designated supervisor, and while this person acts as an agent of the Nursing and Midwifery Council to protect the public, there are many positive benefits for the lifelong learner midwife. The supervisor's role (Nursing and Midwifery Council, 2006d) is broad but it includes:

- acting as a role model
- meeting at least annually with supervisees
- being a resource in implementing change

- encouraging critical evaluation of practice and the use of evidence
- supporting midwives with professional, legal and ethical issues.

The supervisor of midwives must be an experienced exemplary professional and, whilst they will be involved in censuring poor practice, their relationship with supervisees provides a positive opportunity to promote lifelong learning and provide invaluable advice regarding CPD. Qualified midwives should foster a professional relationship with their supervisor.

# Special interests and opportunities

Over the course of pre-registration midwifery or nursing educational experiences, or as your career progresses, you are likely to develop particular interests. Some aspects of care are particularly relevant and are especially interesting. You may become or aspire to become a specialist in your chosen field of practice. A 'special interest' can be almost any aspect of care but the following list gives a few examples:

- breastfeeding
- childhood asthma
- cognitive behavioural therapy in adolescents with eating disorders
- mental health needs of asylum seekers
- nutritional aspects of 'stroke'
- people with learning disabilities and legal processes
- pre-hospital emergency care
- sudden infant death syndrome
- supporting families through Alzheimer's disease
- use of leeches in wound management.

Coinciding with such special interests are client groups which may well have their own representative organizations or associated charities. Some of these organizations share your commitment to the client groups and improvements in care. They aim to disseminate good practice and even to develop expertise amongst nurses and midwives. Their literature, some of which is produced explicitly for health professionals, will provide excellent material to use in your CPD endeavours and you should consider developing good working relationships with selected organizations.

Below is a case study giving insights into how the MS Research Trust may assist nurses in their CPD needs. It provides tangible opportunities for both emerging and established multiple sclerosis specialist nurses.

## MS Research Trust – case study

This is a national charity which aims to provide information, education programmes for health professionals, and research focused on helping people to live with MS (http://www.mstrust.org.uk/default.jsp). For nurses with a special interest in MS it provides the following:

- study days directed at all with an interest in MS
- development module in clinical MS: specialist level
  - an intensive accredited MS module which is rigorously assessed by its associated university; a one-week residential course, bringing together key specialist speakers from a wide range of disciplines
  - aimed at new-in-post MS specialists in the UK, reflecting current NHS initiatives
  - course costs and residential fees, subject to conditions, paid for through sponsorship and the Department of Health as part of their risk-sharing scheme
- master classes providing specialists with an in-depth examination of selected issues such as:
  - transcutaneous electrical nerve stimulation (TENS)
  - Mental Capacity Act 2005
  - depression
  - postural management
- annual conference
- annual two-day course for MS specialist nurses.

# Formal structured learning

Many nurses and midwives will wish to engage in some form of study programme or course and the choice of topics is vast. Many provide interdisciplinary learning environments with opportunities to learn with non-nurses and non-midwives. Study modes also vary considerably, for example:

- blended learning
- distance learning
- e-learning
- in person attendance
- secondment
- self-directed learning.

## Exercise 11.4

- Look at your personal development plan (see Chapter 10) and identify the medium-term goals you have set
- Select one which may require some form of formal study
- Reflect on the possible modes of study outlined above and determine which best suits your needs
- Investigate which organizations could provide both the content and the mode of study you require
- Seriously consider extending your repertoire of delivery modes you are comfortable with
- Discuss this at your next development review meeting or earlier, in time to meet deadlines for course applications

### Example

- You may be a midwife or nurse with two years post-qualifying experience
- You have rotated around three areas of a unit within the same organization
- You have developed good habits which embrace regular lifelong learning activities
- Several critical incidents, some involving clients, others involving students, have occurred in this period
- These have all had ethical dimensions and your reflection has identified your limited knowledge of legal and ethical issues
- You decide that you would like to return to study to satisfy your curiosity and close the perceived knowledge gap
- Exploring what is available you find that:
  - locally there is a taught course, requiring weekly attendance, which is discipline-specific
  - there is a distance learning course supported by multi-media and Internet provisions
  - another institution, based 60 miles away, offers a blended approach with two separate residential weeks of intense study, regular e-contact with lecturers and peers, and clearly mapped out reading assignments
- You prefer taught classroom-based study, but the practical difficulty while working shifts means that a lot of attendance would be inconvenient
- The third option is selected and you negotiate some study leave and plan to book bed and breakfast for three nights to accommodate the residential aspects of the course

# Using information technology to facilitate LLL

It is important that each nurse and each midwife develops regular LLL habits such as those reported by Mottershead (2006), a newly qualified independent midwife who carries out a literature search as a weekly occurrence to support her practice. It is vital that you first have basic IT skills, a characteristic that is associated with an average time saving of an astonishing 39 minutes per day (Information Centre for Health and Social Care, 2005). Your organization may support the European Computer Driving Licence scheme and consider it to represent essential IT skills. If you have identified IT skills deficits then this is a robust training programme which you should explore.

Keeping up-to-date with developments in your subject area can be a time consuming process. You may need to read newspapers and journals, visit websites, conduct literature searches and attend relevant events to maintain your professional portfolio. However, you can save time by utilizing IT to deliver relevant information directly to your computer.

# RSS News Feeds

News Feeds are a way of collating any new information appearing on a website and delivering it to a website called a News Reader where it can be read along with any other News Feeds. Say for instance you are interested in cancer nursing and you regularly visit four websites and read two online journals. With an RSS (Really Simple Syndication) News Feed it is possible to set up your News Reader to download anything added to the websites and the headlines from the latest edition of the online journals. This would allow you to visit one website instead of six!

### Some examples

Information on RSS News Feeds from the BBC News website
http://news.bbc.co.uk/1/hi/help/3223484.stm

An example of a BBC Health News Feed
http://newsrss.bbc.co.uk/rss/newsonline_uk_edition/health/rss.xml

How to set a RSS News Feed to receive articles from BioMed Central
http://www.biomedcentral.com/info/about/rss/

# Blogs

Blogs or weblogs are a form of online diary which allows members to post comments and information that can be read by the rest of the group. If you wished to discuss mental health issues with other professionals you could set up a blog or join an existing one. They are easily found on the Internet and can be set up to download information onto your News Reader.

### Some examples

How to set up a blog for yourself
http://www.blogger.com/start

Some mental health blogs
http://mentalhealth.about.com/od/blogs/Mental_ Health_Blogs.htm

Schizophrenia blog
http://www.schizophrenia.com/sznews/

# Discussion lists

Discussion lists are similar to blogs in that you can post information by e-mail to a central address which will then circulate it to the members via their e-mail accounts. If you wished to keep up-to-date with midwifery, joining a discussion list would enable you to draw on the experience of other midwives across the world.

### Some examples

How to join a discussion list
http://commtechlab.msu.edu/Sites/letsnet/noframes/bigideas/b9/b9u2l6.html

Royal College of Midwives discussion lists
http://www.rcm.org.uk/professional/pages/interact.php?id=1

Birth related discussion lists
http://www.fensende.com/Users/swnymph/email. html

Basic IT skills are increasingly required to facilitate many learning endeavours. At least annually you should make a conscious effort to take stock, review and revise your personal development plan. Using an e-portfolio will help you keep this record live and regularly updated as you frequently check selected Internet facilities.

# Conclusions

It has been the intention of this book to focus on encouraging nurses and midwives and their respective students to develop study skills and so become successful in the process of learning. This process is necessary across all disciplines and levels within nursing and midwifery from novice to expert. Becoming proficient or expert as a learner will provide the necessary tools, strategies, skills and attitude to embrace the ethos of lifelong learning and enable you to make the best use of the CPD opportunities available to you. You may by now be convinced that a commitment to patient and client care requires a commitment to developing your own study skills and in doing so LLL and your professional practice will become more enjoyable and rewarding.

# References

Altun, I. (2003) The perceived problem solving ability and values of student nurses and midwives. *Nurse Education Today*, 23(8): 575–84.

Anon (2001) The increasing impact of ehealth on consumer behaviour. *Healthcare News*, http://www.harrisinteractive.com/news/newsletters/healthnews/HI_Health-CareNews2001Vol1_iss21.pdf (accessed 15 January 2007).

Anon (2004) Rewards on the wards. *Disability Now*, http://www.disabilitynow.org.uk/search/z03_11_No/rewards.shtml (accessed 3 January 2007).

Arthritis Care (2006) *About Arthritis*, http://www.arthritiscare.org.uk/Home (accessed 15 May 2006).

Atkins, S. and Murphy, K. (1994) Reflective practice. *Nursing Standard*, 8(39) 49–56.

Audi, R. (1998) *Epistemology: a Contemporary Introduction to the Theory of Knowledge*. London: Routledge.

Bandura, A. (1977) *Social Learning Theory*. London: Prentice-Hall.

Bartlett, P. (2005) *Blackstone's Guide to the Mental Capacity Act 2005*. Oxford: Oxford University Press.

Basford, L. and Slevin, O. (eds) (1999) *Theory and Practice of Nursing: an Integrated Approach to Patient Care*, 2nd edn. Cheltenham: Stanley Thornes.

Baugh, S.G. and Sullivan, S.E. (2005) Mentoring and career development. *Career Development International*, 10(6/7): 425–8.

Bekhradnia, B., Whitnall, C. and Sastry, T. (2006) *The Academic Experience of Students in English Universities*. London: Higher Education Policy Institute, http://www.hepi.ac.uk/downloads/27Academicexperienceofstudents.pdf (accessed 15 January 2007).

Benner, P. (1984) *From Novice to Expert: Excellence and Power in Clinical Nursing Practice*. Menlo Park: Addison-Wesley.

Bloom, B. (2006) Taxonomy of educational objectives, pp. 100–1. In: M. Tennant (ed.) *Psychology and Adult Learning*, 3rd edn. Abingdon: Routledge.

Brink, P.J. and Wood, M.J. (1988) *Basic Steps in Planning Nursing Research: from Question to Proposal*, 3rd edn. Boston: Jones and Bartlett.

Brown, R. (1995) *Portfolio Development and Profiling for Nurses*, 2nd edn. Dinton: Quay Books.

Bruner, J.S. (1961) The act of discovery. *Harvard Educational Review*, 31(1): 21–32.

Burns, S. and Bulman, C. (eds) (2000) *Reflective Practice in Nursing: the Growth of the Professional Practitioner*, 2nd edn. Oxford: Blackwell Science.

Buzan, T. (1974) *Use Your Head*. London: BBC Books.

Campbell, H., Hotchkiss, R., Bradshaw, N. and Porteous, M. (1998) Integrated care pathways. *British Medical Journal*, 316(7125): 133–7.

Canning, B. and Scullion, P. (2001) Judging evidence using legal concepts. *British Journal of Therapy and Rehabilitation*, 8(6): 206–11.

Canter, D. and Fairbairn, G. (2006) *Becoming an Author: Advice for Academics and other Professionals*. Maidenhead: Open University Press.

Carnwell, R. and Daly, W. (2001) Strategies for the construction of a critical review of the literature. *Nurse Education in Practice*, 1(2): 57–63.

Carr, K.C., Fullerton, J.T., Severino, R. and McHugh, M.K. (1996) Barriers to completion of a nurse-midwifery distance education program. *Journal of Distance Education/Revue de l'enseignement à distance* 11(1), http://cade.athabascau.ca/vol11.1/carretal.html (accessed 15 January 2007).

Castle, A. (2003) Demonstrating critical evaluation skills using Bloom's taxonomy. *International Journal of Therapy and Rehabilitation*, 10(8): 369–73.

Castle, A. (2006) Assessment of the critical thinking skills of student radiographers. *Radiography*, 12(2): 88–95.

Cohen, S., Kessler, R.C. and Gordon, L. (eds) (1997) *Measuring Stress: a Guide for Health and Social Scientists*. Oxford: Oxford University Press.

Cooperstein, S.E., Kocevar-Weidinger, E. (2004) Beyond active learning: a constructivist approach to learning. *Reference Services Review*, 32(2): 141–8, http://www.emeraldinsight.com/10.1108/00907320410537658 (accessed 3 January 2007).

Corr, S., Beaulieu, K. and Griffiths, S. (2006) Research governance, not research 'somtherance'. *International Journal of Therapy and Rehabilitation*, 13(2): 56.

Costa, A. and Kallick, B. (1993) Through the lens of a critical friend. *Educational Leadership*, 51(2): 49–51.

Cottrell, S. (2003) *The Study Skills Handbook*, 2nd edn. Basingstoke: Palgrave Macmillan.

Crowe, M.T. and O'Malley, J. (2006) Teaching critical reflection skills for advanced mental health nursing practice: a deconstructive-reconstructive approach. *Journal of Advanced Nursing*, 56(1): 79–87.

Cutcliffe, J.R. and Ward, M. (2003) *Critiquing Nursing Research*. Dinton: Quay Books.

Day-Stirk, F. (2006) What about the three A's? *Midwives*, 9(10): 372.

Department of Health (1998) *A First Class Service: Quality in the New NHS*. London: The Stationery Office.

Department of Health (2001) *Working Together – Learning Together: Framework for Lifelong Learning for the NHS*. London: DoH, http://www.dh.gov.uk/assetRoot/04/05/88/96/04058896.pdf (accessed 17 January 2007).

Department of Health (2003) *The Essence of Care: Patient-focused Benchmarking for Clinical Governance*. http://195.33.102.76/assetRoot/04/12/79/15/04127915.pdf (accessed 31 July 2006).

Department of Health (2004a) *Patient and Public Involvement in Health: the Evidence for Policy Implementation*. London: DoH, http://www.dh.gov.uk/assetRoot/04/08/23/34/04082334.pdf (accessed 15 January 2007).

Department of Health (2004b) *Learning for Delivery; Making Connections between Post-qualification Learning/Continuing Professional Development and Service Planning*. London: DoH, http://www.dh.gov.uk/assetRoot/04/08/72/20/04087220.pdf (accessed 17 January 2007).

Department of Health (2004c) *Agenda for Change: What Will it Mean for You? A Guide for Staff*.

London: DoH, http://www.dh.gov.uk/assetRoot/04/09/08/59/04090859.pdf (accessed 17 January 2007).

Department of Health (2005) *Research governance framework for health and social care.* (online) 2nd edn. London, Department of Health. Available from http://www.dh.gov.uk/assetRoot/04/12/24/27/04122427.pdf (accessed 16 January 2007).

Department of Health (2006a) *Best Research for Best Health: a New National Health Research Strategy.* London: Department of Health, http://www.dh.gov.uk/assetRoot/04/12/71/52/04127152.pdf (accessed 16 January 2007).

Department of Health (2006b) *Modernising Nursing Careers: Setting the Direction.* London: Department of Health, http://www.dh.gov.uk/assetRoot/04/13/87/57/04138757.pdf (accessed 16 January 2007).

Dochy, F., Segers, M. and Sluijsmans, D. (1999) The use of self, peer and co-assessment in higher education: a review. *Studies in Higher Education,* 14(3): 331–50.

Ely, C. and Lear, D. (2003) The practice learning experience, pp. 14–32. In: S. Glen and P. Parker (eds) *Supporting Learning in Nursing Practice: a Guide for Practitioners.* Basingstoke: Palgrave Macmillan.

Evans, L. and Abbot, I. (1998) *Teaching and Learning in Higher Education.* London: Cassell.

Eysenck, M.W. and Keane, M.T. (2005) *Cognitive Psychology: a Student's Handbook,* 5th edn. Hove: Psychology Press.

Forbes, D. and Spence, J. (1991) An experiment in assessment for a large class. In: R. Smith (ed.) *Innovations in engineering education.* London: Ellis Horwood.

Forrest, S., Risk, I., Masters, H. and Brown, N. (2000) Mental health service user involvement in nurse education: exploring the issues. *Journal of Psychiatric and Mental Health Nursing,* 7(1): 51–7.

Fowler, J. (ed.) (2005) *Staff Nurse Survival Guide: Essential Questions and Answers for the Practising Staff Nurse.* London: Quay Books.

Fullerton, J.T. and Thompson, J.B. (2005) Examining the evidence for the International Confederation of Midwives' essential competencies for midwifery practice. *Midwifery,* 21(1): 2–13.

Gash, S. (1989) *Effective literature searching for research,* 2nd edn. Aldershot: Gower.

Gershaw, D. (1989) *Line on Life.* http://wik.ed.uiuc.edu/index.php/locus_of_control (accessed 15 March 2006).

Gillam, S. and Brooks, F. (eds) (2001) *New Beginnings: Towards Patient and Public Involvement in Primary Healthcare.* London: King's Fund.

Gopee, N. (1999) Referencing academic assignments. *Nursing Standard,* 13(27):37–40.

Gopee, N. (2002) Demonstrating critical analysis in academic assignments. *Nursing Standard,* 16(35): 45–52.

Gopee, N. (2005) Facilitating the implementation of lifelong learning in nursing. *British Journal of Nursing,* 14(14): 761–7.

Graham, H. and Blackburn, C. (1998) The socio-economic patterning of health and smoking behaviour among mothers with young children on income support. *Sociology of Health and Illness,* 20(2): 215–40.

Hart, C. (1998) *Doing a Literature Review: Releasing the Social Science Research Imagination.* London: Sage.

Harvey, L. (2006) What is the student experience anyway? *Academy Exchange,* 14: 14–15.

Hull, C. and Redfern, L. (1996) *Profiles and Portfolios: A Guide for Nurses and Midwives*, 2nd edn. Basingstoke: Palgrave Macmillan.

Information Centre for Health and Social Care (2005) *Basic IT Skills for the NHS: ECDL 'FiT for Purpose' Re-visit*. Leeds: ICHSC, http://www.ic.nhs.uk/informatics/support/ecdl/file (accessed 17 January 2007).

Jackson, K. and Sheldon, L. (2000) Demystifying the academic aura: preparing a poster. *Nurse Researcher*, 7(3): 70–3.

Jarvis, P. (2005) Lifelong education and its relevance to nursing. *Nurse Education Today*, 25(8): 655–60.

Johns, C. (1994) Nuances of reflection. *Journal of Clinical Nursing*, 3(2): 71–5.

Joint Information Systems Committee (2005) *Deterring, Detecting and Dealing with Student Plagiarism*. http://www.jisc.ac.uk/index.cfm?name=pub_plagiarism (accessed 15 January 2007).

Kippen, S. (2003) Teacher reflection and theories of learning online. *Journal of Educational Enquiry*, 4(1): 19–30.

Lincoln, M., Stockhausen, L. and Maloney, D. (1997) Learning processes in clinical education. In: L. McAllister, M. Lincoln, S. McLeod and D. Maloney (eds) *Facilitating Learning in Clinical Settings*. Cheltenham: Stanley Thornes.

London, F. (1999) *No Time to Teach? A Nurse's Guide to Patient and Family Education*. Philadelphia: Lippincott.

Macnee, C.L. and McCabe, S. (2008) *Understanding Nursing Research. Reading and Using Research in Evidence-Based Practice*, 2nd edn. Philadelphia: Lippincott Williams and Wilkins.

Mangena, A. and Chabeli, M.M. (2005) Strategies to overcome obstacles in the facilitation of critical thinking in nursing education. *Nurse Education Today*, 25(4): 291–8.

Martin, G.W. (1996) An approach to the facilitation and assessment of critical thinking in nurse education. *Nurse Education Today*, 16(1): 3–9.

Martin, M.A. (1985) Students' applications of self-questioning study techniques: an investigation of their efficacy. *Reading Psychology*, 6(1–2): 69–83.

Mason, T. and Whitehead, E. (2003) *Thinking Nursing*. Buckingham: Open University Press.

Masterson, A. (2005) Writing skills and developing an argument, pp. 185–208. In: S. Maslin-Prothero (ed.) *Bailliere's Study Skills for Nurses and Midwives*, 3rd edn. Edinburgh: Elsevier.

McAlearney, A.S. (2005) Exploring mentoring and leadership development in healthcare organizations: experience and opportunities. *Career Development International*, 10(6/7): 493–511.

McKenzie, F., White, C.A., Kendall, S., Finlayson, A., Urquhart, M. and Williams, I. (2006) Psychological impact of colostomy pouch change and disposal. *British Journal of Nursing*, 15(6): 308–16.

Melrose, S. (2006) Creating a psychiatric mental health portfolio: an assignment activity that works. *Nurse Education in Practice*, 6(5): 288–94.

Miller, C.M.L. and Parlett, M. (1974) *Up to the Mark: A Study of the Examination Game*. London: Society for Research into Higher Education.

Mottershead, N. (2006) A time of independence. *Midwives*, 9(10): 400–1.

Muir-Gray, J.A. (1997) *Evidence-based Healthcare*. Edinburgh: Churchill Livingstone.

National Committee of Enquiry into Higher Education (1997) *Higher Education in the Learning Society: Main Report.* Report of the National Committee, chairman Sir Ron Dearing. London: The Stationery Office.

National Health Service (2002) *Expert Patients Programme.* http://www.expertpatients. nhs.uk/about.shtml (accessed May 15 2006).

National Health Service, National Library for Health (2005) *Protocols and Care Pathways Specialist Library. Elective Caesarean Section ICP (Incorporating pre-operative assessment),* http://www.library.nhs.uk/pathways/viewResource.aspx?resID=88647&code=14c95344e 35b390033b0dfd7b21ed5ff (accessed 20 May 2006).

Neurological Alliance (2004) *Nero Numbers: a Brief Review of the Numbers of People in the UK with a Neurological Condition.* London: Neurological Alliance, http://www.neural.org.uk/ docs/neuro_numbers/NEURONUM.PDF (accessed 15 January 2007).

Northedge, A. (2005) *The Good Study Guide,* 2nd edn. Milton Keynes: Open University Press.

Northway, R. (2000) Finding out together: lessons in participatory research for the learning disability nurse. *Mental Healthcare,* 31(7): 229–32.

Nursing and Midwifery Council (2002) *A NMC guide for Students of Nursing and Midwifery.* London: Nursing and Midwifery Council, http://www.nmc-uk.org/aFrameDisplay.aspx? DocumentID=1896 (accessed 16 January 2007).

Nursing and Midwifery Council (2004a) *The NMC Code of Professional Conduct: Standards for Conduct, Performance and Ethics.* London: Nursing and Midwifery Council, http://www. nmc-uk.org/aDisplayDocument.aspx?DocumentID=201 (accessed 16 January 2007).

Nursing and Midwifery Council (2004b) *Midwives Rules and Standard.* London: Nursing and Midwifery Council, http://www.nmc-uk.org/aFrameDisplay.aspx?DocumentID=169 (accessed 17 January 2007).

Nursing and Midwifery Council (2006a) *Standards to Support Learning and Assessment in Practice.* London: Nursing and Midwifery Council, http://www.nmc-uk.org/aFrame-Display.aspx?DocumentID=2087 (accessed 24 January 2007).

Nursing and Midwifery Council (2006b) *The PREP Handbook.* London: Nursing and Midwifery Council, http://www.nmc-uk.org/aFrameDisplay.aspx?DocumentID=1636 (accessed 17 January 2007).

Nursing and Midwifery Council (2006c) *Clinical Supervision.* London: Nursing and Midwifery Council, http://www.nmc-uk.org/aFrameDisplay.aspx?DocumentID=1558 (accessed 17 January 2007).

Nursing and Midwifery Council (2006d) *Standards for the Preparation and Practice of Supervisors of Midwives.* London: Nursing and Midwifery Council, http://www.nmc-uk.org/ aFrameDisplay.aspx?DocumentID=2229 (accessed 17 January 2007).

Nursing and Midwifery Order (2001) SI 2002/253. Article 15(1) (b). Norwich: The Stationery Office.

Palmgreen, P. (1984) Uses and gratifications: a theoretical perspective, pp. 61–72. In: R.N. Bostrom (ed.) *Communication Yearbook 8.* London: Sage.

Parkinson's Disease Society (2005) *Competencies: an Integrated Career and Competency Framework for Nurses Working in PD Management.* London: Parkinson's Disease Society.

Pearce, R. (2003) *Profiles and Portfolios of Evidence.* Cheltenham: Nelson Thornes.

Peterson, C., Maier, S.F. and Seligman, M.E.P. (1995) *Learned Helplessness: a Theory for the Age of Personal Control,* 2nd edn. New York: Oxford University Press.

Phillips, E.M. and Pugh, D.S. (2005) *How to Get a PhD: a Handbook for Students and their Supervisors*, 4th edn. Maidenhead: Open University Press.

Polit-O'Hara, D.F. and Beck, C.T. (2006) *Essentials of Nursing Research: Methods, Appraisal, and Utilization*, 6th edn. Philadelphia: Lippincott Williams and Wilkins.

Pollard, C. and Hibbert, C. (2004) Expanding student learning using patient pathways. *Nursing Standard*, 19(2): 40–3.

Price, B. (2005) Self-assessment and reflection in nurse education. *Nursing Standard*, 19(29): 33–7.

Punch, K.F. (2000) *Developing Effective Research Proposals*. London: Sage.

Quinn, F.M. (2000) *Principles and Practice of Nurse Education*, 4th edn. Cheltenham: Stanley Thornes.

Race, P. and Brown, S. (2001) *The Lecturers Toolkit*, 2nd edn. London: Kogan Page.

Redman, P. (2006) *Good Essay Writing: a Social Sciences Guide*, 3rd edn. London: Open University Press in association with Sage Publications.

Rees, C. (1997) *An Introduction to Research for Midwives*, 2nd edn. Hale: Books for Midwives Press.

Robins, S. and Mayer, R.E. (1993) Schema training in analogical reasoning. *Journal of Educational Psychology*, 85(3): 529–38.

Robson, C. (2006) Evaluation research, pp. 289–301. In: K. Gerrish and A. Lacey (eds) *The Research Process in Nursing*, 5th edn. Oxford: Blackwell Publishing.

Rowntree, D. (1977) *Assessing Students: How Shall we Know Them?* London: Harper & Row.

Rowntree, D. (1998) *Learn How to Study: a Realistic Approach*, 4th edn. London: Warner Books.

Royal College of Midwives (2006) *Learning: Continuing Professional Development Programme*. London: Royal College of Midwives, http://www.rcm.org.uk/professional/pages/learning.php?id=1 (accessed 17 January 2007).

Royal College of Nursing (2004) *The Future Nurse: Trends and Predictions for the Nurse Workforce*. London: Royal College of Nursing, http://www.rcn.org.uk/downloads/futurenurse/fn-trends.doc (accessed 15 January 2007).

Royal College of Nursing (2006) *Discussing and Preparing Evidence at your First Personal Development Review: Guidance for RCN Members on the NHS Knowledge and Skills Framework*. London: Royal College of Nursing, http://www.rcn.org.uk/publications/pdf/rcn_k_s_2006.pdf (accessed 17 January 2007).

Scheffer, B.K., Rubenfeld, M.G. (2000) Consensus statement on critical thinking in nursing. *Journal of Nursing Education*, 39(8): 352–9.

Scottish Executive, Student Awards Agency for Scotland (2006) *Disabled Students Allowance*. Edinburgh: Scottish Executive, http://www.student-support-saas.gov.uk/disabled.htm (accessed 3 January 2007).

Scullion, P. (2000) Is the research necessary? Equipoise and other fundamental ethical considerations. *NT Research*, 5(6): 461–9.

Scullion, P. (2003) The decisions and dilemmas of dysphagia management. *International Journal of Therapy and Rehabilitation*, 10(5): 192.

Shorten, A. and Wallace, M.C. (2001) Developing information literacy: a key to evidence based nursing. International Nursing Review, 48(2): 86–92.

Stone, P.W. (2002) Popping the PICO question in research and evidence based practice. *Applied Nursing Research*, 15(3): 197–8.

Surgenor, L.J., Horn,J., Hudson, S.M., Lunt, H. and Tennent, J. (2000) Metabolic control and psychological sense of control in women with diabetes mellitus. Alternative considerations of the relationship. *Journal of Psychosomatic Research*, 49(4): 267–73.

Tang, C. (1994) Assessment and student learning: effects of modes of assessment on students' preparation strategies, pp. 151–170. In: G. Gibbs (ed.) *Improving Student Learning: Theory and Practice*. Oxford: Oxford Brookes University, The Oxford Centre for Staff Development.

Terry, J. (N.D.) *'Moving On': a Package of Information and Workshop Materials Addressing Skills for Higher Education, to Assist in Building Confidence and Success*. Collaborative Widening Participation Project (Coventry University, University College Worcester, The University of Warwick), http://www.dcs.warwick.ac.uk/undergraduate/movingon/0.pdf (accessed 3 January 2007).

United Kingdom Central Council for Nursing Midwifery and Health Visiting (UKCC) (1986) *Project 2000: a New Preparation for Practice*. London: UKCC.

United Kingdom Central Council for Nursing Midwifery and Health Visiting (UKCC) (1999) *Fitness for Practice*. The UK Commission for Nursing and Midwifery Education, Chair Sir Leonard Peach. London: UKCC.

University of Sussex, Sussex Language Institute (N.D.) *Critical Analysis, Argument and Opinion*. http://www.sussex.ac.uk/languages/1–6–8–2–3.html (accessed 10 November 2006).

University of York, Centre for Reviews and Dissemination (2006) ABOUT CRD. York: University of York, http://www.york.ac.uk/inst/crd/aboutcrd.htm (accessed 9 June 2006).

Walters, J. and Adams, J. (2002) A child health nursing objective structured clinical examination (OSCE). *Nurse Education in Practice*, 2(4): 224–9.

Watling, R., Hopkins, D., Harris, A. and Beresford, J. (1998) Between the devil and the deep blue sea? Implications for school and LEA development following an accelerated inspection programme. In L. Stoll and K. Myers (eds) *No Quick Fixes: Perspectives on Schools in Difficulty*. London: Falmer Press.

Watson, R., Wray, J., Stimpson, A., Gibson, H., Aspland, J. and Carrison, J. (2006) *'A Wealth of Knowledge': the Employment Experiences of Older Nurses, Midwives and the NHS*. Hull: Faculty of Health and Social Care, University Of Hull, http://www.hull.ac.uk/on/documents/FinalReport_000.pdf (accessed 15 January 2007).

Welsh Rural Postgraduate Unit and Local Health Board Powys (N.D.) *Protected Learning Time in Powys, Programme Framework*. Newtown: Institute of Rural Health, http://www.rural-health.ac.uk/ftpdownloads/PLT%20framework.pdf (accessed 17 January 2007).

Welsh, M.M. (2006) Engaging with peer assessment in post-registration nurse education. *Nurse Education in Practice*, 7(2): 75–81.

White, E. (2006) Devoting time for continuing professional development. *International Journal of Therapy and Rehabilitation*, 13(10): 440.

Wilcox, A. (2005) How to succeed as a lifelong learner. *Primary Healthcare*, 15(10): 43–50.

Wilkie, K. (2000) The nature of problem-based learning, pp. 11–36. In: S. Glen and K. Wilkie (eds) *Problem-Based Learning in Nursing: a New Model for a New Context?* Basingstoke: Macmillan Press.

Wright, D. (1999) HCP (Healthcare Professionals with Disability). *Disability*, http://www.david-j-wright.staff.shef.ac.uk/HCP-disability/index.html (accessed 3 January 2007).

# Glossary

**Academic supervision**   Input to studies provided by a member of the academic staff (supervisor), providing guidance, challenge and supervision often for a designated piece of coursework or research

**Colostomy**   Surgical formation of an artificial anus by connecting the colon (large intestine) to an opening in the abdominal wall

**Course plan**   Document usually provided at the beginning of a course showing an outline of the planned educational experiences, placements, modules and key dates, holiday and completion etc. Usually published in a course handbook, that contains comprehensive information about the course

**Deaf**   Written always with capital 'D' this implies a community comprising those deaf and hard-of-hearing people who share a common language, common experiences and values

**Dissertation**   Comprehensive written study of a specialised subject; substantial academic paper written on an original topic of research, usually presented as one of the final requirements for a doctorate

**e-Learning**   Learning facilitated and supported through the use of information and communications technology; can cover a spectrum of activities from supported learning, to blended learning, to learning that is entirely online

**Equipoise**   State of intellectual equilibrium or balance; being equally poised between options; genuine uncertainty

**Freshers' Week**   The week when new first-year undergraduate students commence a course; often has a timetable which combines orientation to the university, introduction to the course and social events

**Hypothesis**   Tentative statement predicting a relationship between variables, the truth of which is thereupon subject to investigation by appropriate research methods

**Induction Day**   Equates with Freshers' Week; introduces CPD students to life and study at university

**Learning outcome**   Statement often set by lecturers and course planners which defines the intentions of a learning experience in terms of the expected results. It is applied to courses, modules and other educational events e.g. lecture or conference presentation

**Mindset**   Fixed mental attitude or disposition that predetermines a person's responses to and interpretations of situations; an inclination or habit of thinking

**Mission statement**   Core purpose of an organization, why it exists, an organization's description of itself, the declaration of values, goals, and aspirations; the organization's unique sense of direction

**Natural language**   In database searching, a natural language search allows the user to type common words and phrases as a search strategy. Natural language searching often retrieves irrelevant results compared with 'controlled vocabulary' (subject headings) searching

**NMC**   Nursing and Midwifery Council, the UK organization which has statutory responsibility for protecting the public by maintaining a register, ensuring standards are set and maintained and investigating practitioners when required

**ODP**   Operating department practitioner, a relatively new professional group, governed by the Health Professions Council; practitioners work in anaesthetics and other aspects of operating theatres

**Oncology**   Scientific study of the physical, chemical, and biological properties, features and treatment of cancers. This is a recognized specialism within medicine and nursing

**Ornithologist**   Specialist in the scientific study of birds, the term is often applied to people who do this as a hobby ('twitcher')

**Pebble pad**   Trademark of software which includes an electronic portfolio. It is offered via some universities and may then be used after completion of a course

**Respondent validation**   Technique commonly used in qualitative types of research where the initial analysis, e.g. of interview data, is returned to the individual who was interviewed (the respondent) to get them to check for accuracy (validate)

**Sim man**   Short for 'simulation man', a full-size model of a human being used by health professionals to learn and develop clinical skills. It uses computer technology to generate appropriate responses to stimuli applied during training, making it realistic and stressful during training periods. Normally found in skills laboratories, mock-up intensive care units and other training facilities

**Skills laboratory**   Designated well-equipped room for teaching and learning practical skills required in health care. Practice under close supervision is facilitated sometimes using 'volunteer patients'

**Supernumerary status**   Not being counted as one of the regular members of a group or team. In clinical placement this implies not being counted as a member of the *workforce* since the student is primarily on placement to learn

**Superscript**   Symbol or character that appears slightly above a line in a body of text; in academic referencing used in the Vancouver system where references are listed in numeric order at the end of the text

**Theologian**   Specialist in theology, the study of God and of God's relation to the world

**Trigger**   Something such as a word, a question, an object or an experience used as a stimulus resulting in a response; used in 'problem-based learning' triggers are deliberately presented to stimulate learning

**URL**   Uniform resource locator, a string of characters used to represent and identify a page of information on the World Wide Web; the web address e.g. http://www.yourwebpage.co.uk

**Variables**   Quantity that may assume any one of a set of values, a measurable factor in data collection, e.g. stress level, number of hospital admissions for individual patients; things which may vary

**Web browser**   Program used to access the Internet services and resources available through the World Wide Web. There are various web browsers; the university will have one of preference installed on its computers. Examples include Netscape, Firefox, Internet Explorer

**Web CT**   Web Course Tools; an online proprietary virtual learning environment system which is used extensively in many universities for e-learning. Lecturers can add to their course tools discussion boards, mail systems and live chat, along with content such as documents and links to web pages

# Index

Academic supervision, 172, 216
Accountability, 90, 185, 202
Action plan, 85, 93, 160
Action plan for CPD, 200
Active learning, 59–60
Active reading strategy, 65
Acts of Parliament, 45–6
Adjacency searching, 112
Adkins and Murphy model of reflection, 94
Agenda for change, 192, 201
Analysis *see* Critical analysis
AND (Boolean operator), 111
Approaches to study, 13–18
Argument, development of, 70–5, 149
  *see also* Critical thinking
Assessment 104, 136,
  criteria for, 153, 165
  failure, 179–80
  formative, 163–4
  methods of, 173–7
  planning for success in, 172–3
  practice, 164
  preparing for 167, 170, 172
  self, 163
  summative, 163–4
  types of, 162–4
  value of, 162–3
Assessment criteria for books, 44–5
Assessment criteria for websites, 49
Assessor 86, 163
Athens authentication, 41
  *see also* Passwords
Atkins, S., 95
Attitude to learning, 58–9

Behaviour, 11
Bibliographic database, 47
Bibliographic reference software, 117–18
Bibliography, 20, 74
Blog, 207
Bloom, B., 148–9
Bloom's Taxonomy, 149
Books
  assessment criteria for, 44–5
  contents page, 62
  index to, 63
  parts of, 61–2
  reference to, 42
Boolean operators, 111
Broadband internet connection, 30

Care pathway, 86–7
Career
  development, 84, 188, 203
  plan, 185
  mentor, 187
Castle, A. 150., 151, 153
Catalogue, library, 43
Cheating, 19, 27; *see also* Plagiarism
CINAHL subject headings, 108
Citation searching, 115–16
Citations in-text, 20, 75
Clinical supervision, 201–2
Cognitive learning, 148, 150
Cognitive levels, 148–9, 155
Collusion, 19, 27
  *see also* Plagiarism
Communication skills, 12, 19, 81, 89, 91, 169
Computers *see* Information technology
Concerns about course, 8–9

Confidence 11, 28, 96, 154, 185
Confidentiality of patients, learner's
    obligation to, 82–4
Consensus formation, 129
Continuous Professional Development
    *see* CPD
    *see also* PREP
Contributing to learning, 10–11
Control
    emotional, 27
    locus of, 24
Coping with practice, 96–7
Cornell system of note taking, 68
Course plan, 33, 216
CPD, 96, 165, 187, 193–4, 198
    action plan for, 200
    defined, 192
    individual factors, 200
    midwives, 202–3
    organisational factors, 199
    prep standards, 194–5
    socio-political factors, 199
Criteria for assessment, 153, 165
Critical analysis
    concept of, 146
    developing skills in, 153–8
    framework of, 155
    need for, 150–1
Critical evaluation, 127, 152, 155
Critical friend, 26
Critical incident analysis, 92
Critical reflection, 150, 152
Critical thinking, 152–4
Critiquing research, 135–8, 140–1, 152
Cue-consciousness, 170–1
Curriculum vitae, 96

Data storage, 51
Databases, 46–7
Department of Health, 82, 87, 102, 125,
    188, 191, 192–4, 199
Dewey decimal classification, 39–40
Disability and learning, 60–1
Discussion lists, 207
Dissertations, 47, 103, 176–7, 216
Dyslexia, 10, 60

EBP *see* Evidence based practice
Educational experiences *see* Teaching
    methods
E-learning, 216
Emotional resilience, 96–8
Engagement, 12, 20, 98
Equipoise, 138, 216
Essay,
    checking the draft, 76
    parts of, 74
Essay writing *see* Writing
Ethical practice, 123
Evaluating search results, 115–16
Evaluation, *see* Critical evaluation
Evidence
    nature of, 122–4, 126, 135, 168–9
    strength of, 73, 122–5, 134–5
    *see also* Critiquing research
Evidence based practice, 103, 120–2, 128,
    146, 150, 151
    context of, 122–3
Examinations 162–3, 171, 174–5
    marking criteria, 165
    special circumstance, 178
    *see also* Assessments
Expert patients, 81–2

Feedback
    from assessment, 163–6
    from essay, 151
    from failed assignment, 179–80
    from mentor, 85
    sheet, 166
Field searching, databases, 110
File management, 51
Formal debates, 17
Formative assessment, 163–4
Friendships, 7, 10, 25–6
    *see also* Critical friend
Full text database, 47

Goals, 29
Google Scholar (search engine), 48
Gopee, N., 19, 150, 153, 155, 195
Gopee's seven stage framework,
    155–8

Group
  friendship 7,
  work, 8–10, 25, 171
  learning, 11, 13, 25–6, 160
  problem based learning, 16
  representatives, 18–19
  seminar, 14
  support, 180, 186, 200
  virtual, 16, 207
Guided study, 17

Harvard reference style, 19–20
  See also Vancouver reference style
Helplessness, 24
Hierarchy of evidence, 126, 133

Ice-breakers, 7–8
Induction day see Orientation
  programme
Information technology, 37–8, 51, 206
Information, role of, 37
Inter-professional, 86, 88, 151
In-text citations, 20, 75
Intute (medical search engine), 48

Johns, C., 93, 94
Johns model of reflection, 94
Journal reference, 42
Journals, 45

Keyword searching, 109
Knowledge and skills framework, 192

Learning
  active, 59–60
  approaches to, 34
  cognitive, 59, 71, 148, 150
  deep, 34
  definition of, 58–9
  disability and, 60–1
  formal (structured), 204–5
  informal (unstructured), 195, 197–8
  novice, 5–6, 96
  objectives, 85, 148
  outcomes, 23, 87
  pathway, 87–8

  practice, 58, 79–80, 86–8, 92
  process, 5, 17, 20, 22, 57, 58, 148, 193,
    208
  protected time for, 198–9
  reflective, 93
  strategies, 58–9, 92
  surface, 34
  syndicate, 26
  subject / content, 5, 17, 20, 43, 47, 108
Learning disability nursing, 82, 115, 200
Lecture, 14, 67–9, 148
Library, catalogue, 43
Library, use of, 38–41
Library of Congress classification, 39–40
Life experiences, 11, 88
Lifelong learning
  concept examined, 192–3
  context of, 191–2
  definition of, 191
  for midwives, 202–3
  framework of, 195–6, 199–200
  organisations, 199
  reflection on, 80
Listening, 66–7
Literature review, 130, 134, 137–8
  marking guide for, 168–9
  stages in, 134–5
Literature search, aims of, 104
  see also Search
Locus of control, 24

Marking criteria for examinations, 165
Marking guide for a literature review,
    168–9
Memory, 59–60, 83
Mental health nursing, 60, 150
Mentor
  career, 187
  in practice, 84–5
MeSH (Medical Subject Headings), 108
Methods of assessment, 173–7
Microsoft Office (software), 50
Midwifery, 150, 186, 188
Midwives
  supervision of, 202–3
  lifelong learning for, 207

Mind maps, 68–9
Models of reflection, 93–5
Monograph, 44
Motivation, 28

Nested searches, 112–13
Networking, 189, 200
NMC, 95, 185, 217
  code of conduct, 11, 123
  guidance for learners, 82–3, 92
  guidance for mentors, 84–5
  PREP requirements, 194–5
  midwifery, 202–3
Note taking, 66–8
NOT (Boolean operator), 111
Novice learner, 5–6, 96
Nursing and Midwifery Council see NMC

Official publications, 45–6
Online resources, 41–2, 206–7
OPAC (Online Public Access Catalogue),
  42
OR (Boolean operator), 111
Orientation programme, 9, 186–7, 216
OSCE, 173–4

Parkinsons' Law, 33
Parts of an essay, 74
Passwords, 41
  see also Athens authentication
Pathway
  care, 86–7
  learning, 87–8
Patients
  as experts, 81–2
  as teachers, 80–1
  right to confidentiality, 82–4
Pebble pad (software), 96, 217
Personal bibliographic software, 118
Personal development plan, 184, 201,
  205
Personal issues 11, 17, 28, 88, 90, 154,
  157, 178–9, 195–6
PICO, use in searching, 105–6
Placement pathways, 87
Plagiarism, 19, 27, 177

Portfolio, professional, 95–6
Poster presentation, 14, 176, 197
Post Registration Education and Practice
  see PREP
Practice
  assessment 164,
  coping with, 96–7
  ethical, 123
  improvement, 129, 131
  learning from, 58, 79–80, 86–8, 92
  links to theory 83, 174,
  placement, 40, 79, 84–6
  reflective, 89–90
Preceptorship in lifelong learning, 201
PREP, 194–8
Preparing for assessment 166, 170, 172
Prioritising your time, 31–2, 178
Problem based learning, 16
Professional development 22, 89, 163
  see also CPD
Professional portfolio, 95–6
  see also CPD
Professional practice, 25
  accountability, 185
Proof reading, 172–3
Protected learning time, 198–9

Qualifying, transition period, 159, 185–6,
  201
Qualitative research, 125, 128, 139–40
Quantitative research, 125, 128, 137, 139
Quotations, 20, 75

RCM see Royal College of Midwives
RCN see Royal College of Nursing
Reading
  active, 65
  books, 61–3
  list, 41–2
  scanning, 64
  skimming, 64
  speed, 64
  SQ3R, 65–6
  strategies, 61, 63–6
  see also Note taking
Recording search results, 117–18

Reference list *see* Reading list
References, 42
Referencing, 19–20, 76
Reflection
   concept of, 89–92
   critical, 150, 152
   definition, 90
   learning strategy, 57, 92
   models, 93–5
Reflective practice, 89–90
Registering on a course, 7
Registering with the NMC, 185, 192,
   194
Regulations, 11, 175, 177, 179
Relationships, 7, 12, 25–6, 171, 185, 187
   in practice, 85–6
   within organisations, 203
Reliability, 139
Research, 45, 102, 105, 116, 176
   classifications of, 127
   critiquing, 135–8, 140–1, 152
   descriptive, 127
   design, 130–3
   evaluative, 127, 129
   explanatory, 127
   hierarchies, 125
   purpose of, 127, 129
   qualitative, 125, 128, 139–40
   quantitative, 125, 128, 137, 139
   strategy, 125–6
   systematic reviews of, 134
   triangulation, 122
   use of, 123
   validity, 137, 139
Resources for study, 29–30
Revision, 33, 67, 164, 171–2, 186
   classes for 180,
Role-play, 15
Rowntree, D., 22, 58, 175
Royal College of Midwives, 41, 46, 189,
   202, 207
Royal College of Nursing, 10, 41, 46, 189,
   200–1
RSS news feeds, 206

Scanning, reading strategy, 64

Search
   adjacency, 112
   Boolean operators, 111
   citation, 116
   engines, 47–8
   history, 114–15
   keeping records, 117–18
   limits, 113–14
   nested, 112–13
   results, evaluation of, 115–16
   strategy, 104
   terminology, 106–13
   truncation used in, 111
   wildcards used in, 112
   *see also* Literature search
Searching the catalogue, 43–4
Self-motivation, 11
Seminars, 14
Simulation, 17
Skills laboratory, 217
SMART learners, 35
Specialist Practice, 188, 203–4
Spyware, worms and viruses,
   51
Stress, 27, 175, 178, 185
Student services at university, 9,
   180
Student support *see* Support
Study
   buddy, 25–6
   modes, 204
   resources for, 29–30
   timetable, 33–5
Subject headings, 108
Summative assessment, 163–4
Supervision
   academic, 172, 216
   clinical, 201–2
   midwives, 202–3
Support, 10, 15, 25–6, 31, 60–1, 79,
   84–6, 90, 97, 164, 178–80,
   185–6
   organisational, 191–3, 198, 201
   *see also* Clinical supervision
Survival, 97
Syndicate learning, 26–7

Synthesis, 134, 149–50, 153, 155, 165, 168

Systematic reviews, 134

Task analysis, 71–2
Teaching by patients, 80–1
Teaching methods, 12–18
Textbook, 44
Theory - practice links 83, 174
Thesis, 73–4
Time
   capturing, 30
   disposable, 31–2
   management of, 23, 30–5, 66, 177
   protected learning, 198–9
   study timetable, 32–3
Transferable skills, 10, 134
Transition from student to professional, 185–6
Triggers to learning 80, 218
   *see also* Problem based learning
Truncation used in searching, 111
Tutorials, 15

Types of assessment, 162–4

University student services, 9, 180
Validity of research, 137, 138
Vancouver reference style, 20
   *see also* Harvard reference style
Viruses, worms and spyware, 51
Viva, 154, 176

Web based learning, 16
Web log *see* Blog
Website assessment criteria, 49
Wildcards, used in database searches, 112
Worms, viruses and spyware, 51
Writing
   academic conventions for, 70–1
   argument, components of, 73
   assessment of, 73
   essays, 19, 37–8, 70–6
   reflective, 70
   task analysis, 71–2
   thesis, development of, 74–5